EVIDENCE-BASED STRATEGIES IN HERBAL MEDICINE, PSYCHIATRIC DISORDERS AND EMERGENCY MEDICINE

Edited by **Farid A. Badria**

Evidence-based Strategies in Herbal Medicine, Psychiatric Disorders and Emergency Medicine
http://dx.doi.org/10.5772/58511
Edited by Farid A. Badria

Contributors

Tomas Janota, Haque Sh.Nizamie@gmail.Com, Abdulghani Mohamed Alsamarai, Farid A. Badria

Published by InTech

Janeza Trdine 9, 51000 Rijeka, Croatia

Publishing Process Manager Danijela Duric

Technical Editor InTech DTP team

Cover InTech Design team

First published February, 2015

Printed in Croatia

Additional hard copies can be obtained from orders@intechopen.com

Evidence-based Strategies in Herbal Medicine, Psychiatric Disorders and Emergency Medicine, Edited by Farid A. Badria

p. cm.

ISBN 978-953-51-1735-3

For EU product safety concerns:
IN TECH d.o.o., Prolaz Marije Krucifikse Kozulić 3, 51000 Rijeka, Croatia,
info@intechopen.com or visit our website at intechopen.com.

Meet the editor

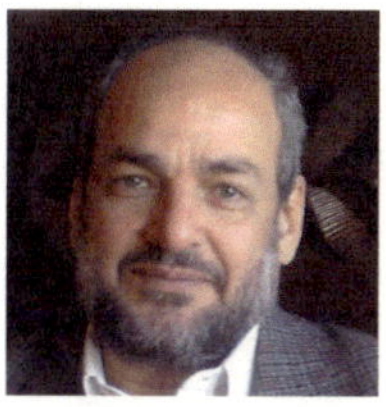

Professor Farid A. Badria, Ph.D. in Pharmacognosy (Microbial Transformation) from the University of Mississippi, USA, with a B.Sc. in Pharmaceutical Sciences, and 2 Masters of Science from Mansoura University and the University of Minnesota.TWAS-Prize (2013), World Intellectual Property Organization Gold Medal, 2011[the best Inventor in Egypt]; State Recognition Outstanding Award in Medicine (Egyptian Academy of Science) 2001; Outstanding Arab Scholar, Kuwait (2000); Khawarazmi International Award, Iran (2000), are just to mention some of the awards he received.
He's also been a scholar of: the Arab Development Fund, Kuwait (2000); ICRO-UNESCO, Chile (1999); UNESCO Biotechnology Fellowship, France (1994); Honorary Fellowship, University of Mississippi, USA (1987-90). Prof. Badria has submitted 44 patents to the Egyptian Academy of Sciences and one to WIPO, of which 17 had been granted final certificates. With over 128 publications, he continues to lead research projects on: developing new therapy for liver dis-orders, immunity, skin disorders, and biomarkers for cancer.

Contents

Preface

Pharmacotherapy is frequently combined with other treatment methods, such as physical therapy and dietotherapy. Drugs are often used in various combinations.

The main objectives in writing this book are to strike a balance between developments in Pharmacotherapy research and the facts that researchers must absorb, and to link scientific advances with clinical practice so that the management of diseases can be based on sound physiological concepts.

The book focuses on three major areas;

Experimental, Preclinical, and Clinical Applications of Herbal Medicine,

Evidence-based strategies in Emergency Medicine

New Approach In Management of psychiatric disorders

The first three chapters describe new and modern applications of common herbs for treatment of several inflammatory and skin disorders e.g. ulcerative colitis, bronchial asthma, osteoarthritis, multiple sclerosis, and melasma. Chapter four deals with severest hypertensive states pose an immediate threat to life and how to manage these situations.

Chapter five is dedicated to tackle polypharmacy psychiatric disorders.

It is our hope that this book may motivate readers to approach the evidence on Pharmacotherapy with an open mind, and thereby spark an interest in making further contributions to the current scientific debate and treatment development efforts.

Farid A. Badria, Ph.D
Professor of Pharmacognosy
Head of Liver Research Lab
Head of Drug Discovery Unit
Faculty of Pharmacy, Mansoura University
Mansoura, Egypt

Section 1

Experimental, Preclinical, and Clinical Applications of Herbal Medicine

Chapter 1

Frankincense (Heaven's Gift) — Chemistry, Biology, and Clinical Applications

Farid A. Badria

Additional information is available at the end of the chapter

http://dx.doi.org/10.5772/59006

1. Introduction

Frankincense, gold, and myrrh were the three gifts from the wise men (the Magi, or the three kings) brought from the East to celebrate the birth of baby Jesus Christ (Bible, Matthew 2:11) According to the Christian belief (Botros et.al. 2003). Nine compounds with immunostimulant and antiviral activity were isolated from the oleogum resin of frankincense (*Boswellia carterii* Birdwood). The frankincense essential oil (3%) found to contain monoterpenes (13.1 %), sesquiterpenes (1 %), and diterpenes (42.5 %). Both isolated oil and resins exhibited strong immunostimulant activity. Badria et al. (2003) proved that the of boswellia, curcumin, and glycyrrhizin exhibited the highest activity against *Herpes simplex* virus. However, boswellia extract retained a significant increase in both FEV1 and PEFR ($P \leq 0.05$ and ≤ 0.01 respectively) with no significant change in FVC in the severe persistent bronchial asthma (Badria et. al. 2003). Boswellia-Curcumin preparation was investigated clinically for treatment of knee osteoarthirits (Badria et. al. 2002). Meanwhile, glycyrrhizin, curcumin and *Boswellia carterii* formula exhibited a hepatoprotective effect and used as endogenous interferon inducer, demonstrating that two phases of the induction of IFN in serum takes place; the induced IFN was regarded as IFN-γ. This induction may be followed by activation of macrophages and augmentation of natural killer (NK) activity through the action of the induced IFN (Badria 2001). This combination was successfully tried in a clinical study as endogenous interferon inducer for treatment of hepatitis C (Badria 2001).

1.1. Historical Background and Folkloric use (Ryman, 1997)

The earliest recorded use of frankincense is found in an inscription on the tomb of a 15th century BC Egyptian queen named Hathsepsut who exported it from Punt's Land "Somalia" to prepare her cosmetics, skin care lotions, and perfumes. Ancient Egyptians burned frankincense as incense in religious ceremonies and rituals. They used it also in embalming and mummification of dead bodies. As an evidence for incense burning, burners with a shape of long handle spoon from the old kingdom in ancient Egypt have been found in which the resin was burnt to provide aromatic warmth on the braziers of their homes in chilly weather. The ancient Egyptians used to grind the resin after charring to provide the black powder that called "Kohl" which used in manufacturing of distinctive eyeliner as seen in a lot of Egyptian art figures. This is the cause of employment of frankincense in the worship of the Egyptian sun God "Horus", a primordial symbol for who was the sacred "All-seeing" eye that burned with judgment.

The use of resin as incense was not confined to ancient Egyptians but extended to Babylonians, Greeks, Romans and Assyrians. It was Herodotus who reported that "in ancient Babylon, 1000 talents weight was offered every year during the feast of Bel, on the great altar of his temple". Nero burnt frankincense by the ton. Romans burnt large quantities of the resin along the routes of the Roman triumphs or victory parades.

The frankincense was a kings' gift, it is said that the queen of Sheba presented a large amount of frankincense, brought by her from Yemen, to the wise King Solomon in 1950 B.C. The original use of the word "incense" was to descripe the aromatic smoke that produced from a substance upon burning, the term has been gradually limited now to frankincense. Interestingly, several myths surrounded the harvest of frankincense; it was believed that valleys where frankincense is collected were guarded by huge horrible winged creatures and red poisonous snakes that attack any one trying to touch the frankincense tree. These mysterious stories tells also that the mythological bird Phoenix, when ready to die, makes its final nest from frankincense and *Cassia* and there; its spirit ascends to the heavens with the perfume of this sacred herb (Miller and Morris, 1988).

The use of camels in transport flourished frankincense trade in the 11th century BC. One of the oldest international trade routes, the frankincense route, runs parallel to the Red Sea outseting from Yemen through a distance of almost 3,400 Km towards Palestine. Such huge trade made Pliny the Elder, the first century Greek Writer, to claim that "the control of the frankincense trade had made the South Arabians the richest people on earth".

Frankincense is one of the crude drugs that are heavily associated with religious rituals and cults; it was thought that incense smokes carried the prayers to the heaven. In Judaism, frankincense was one of the four sweet scents used in compounding the ceremonial incense of Jewish temples. As a part of the meet offering as well as the chew-bread on Sabbath day, pure frankincense was utilized. It was preserved with many other spices in great chamber of the GOD house at Jerusalem.

In Christianity, Frankincense occupied a distinguished place; it was mentioned 22 times in the Bible. According to the Christian belief; gold, frankincense, and myrrh were the three gifts from the wise men (the Magi, or the three kings) brought from the East to celebrate the birth of baby Jesus Christ (Bible, Matthew 2:11). Frankincense enters into the composition of incense now used in the Christian churches.

Frankincense was one of the most prized and costly substance in the ancient world, worth more than its weight in gold. Dioscorides and others mentioned the therapeutic use of the resin

http://dx.doi.org/10.5772/59006

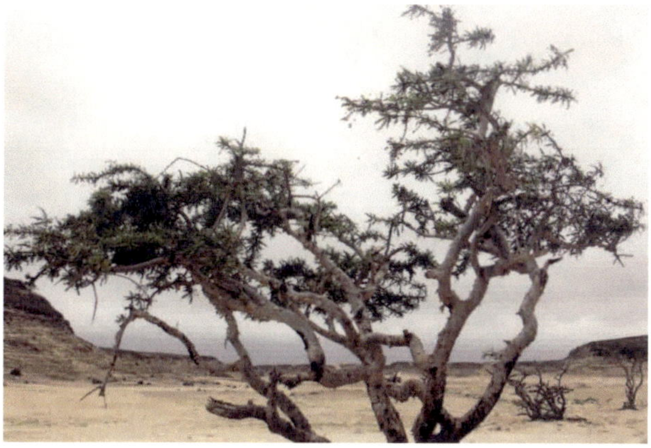

Figure 1. *Boswellia carterii* Birdwood Tree; Frankincense

in the treatment of skin disorders, in ophthalmology, hemorrhages and pneumonia. Pliny the Elder (1st century) mentions it as antidote to hemlock (Encyclopedia Britannica web site). The Iranian physician Avicenna "Ibn Sina" (10 th century) in his book "El-Kanon Fi El-Tibb" thought that frankincense was useful in many disorders and disease as fever, gastric disorders and tumors. *B. carterii* is used almost for everything in China.. In Ayurvedic medicine (Kapoor, 1990) the resin is prescribed in chronic lung diseases, diarrhea, dysentery, pulmonary diseases, menorrhea, dysmenorrhea, syphilis, piles, and liver disorders. The oil extracted from the gum resin is prescribed with a demulcent drink in gonorrhea. A paste made of the gum resin with coconut oil or lemon juice is applied to ulcers, swellings, boils, and ringworm (Chopra *et al.*, 1956). The antiseptic action of the resin encourages healing so it is used to treat ulcers and wounds. The resin is used nowadays in manufacture of incense, and as ingredient in plasters and fumigating pastilles (Wallis, 1967). It is also important as a scent and a fixative in perfumery industry. The recommended dosage of frankincense in inflammatory or bronchoconstrictive conditions is 400 mg three times daily. The frankincense is one of the safest herbals. Toxicity studies of *Boswellia* in rats and primates showed that LD_{50} was established at more than 2 g/kg (Murray, 1995).

Frankincense is an oleogum resin obtained through a deep longitudinal incision the trunk of the Boswellia tree.The milk-like juice which exudes is hardened by exposure to the air. In about three months, the resin attains the required degree of consistency, hardening into yellowish tears (Fig. 2). (Miller and Morris, 1988).

Even the frankincense collected from the wounds is graded into several grades (Singh and Atal, 1988) of which are, Grade I (Tears); which is the best and most carefully selected grade of white color; Grade II (Reddish) that is mixed white and reddish quality which contains some particles of the bark; and Grade III (Dust and Sifting). The latter grade, because of its low price and finer size, is the most suitable quality for distillation of volatile oil. The harvest lasts from May till the middle of September, when the first shower of monsoon rain puts a close to the gathering for that year. Once the collection season is completed, the raw frankincense is allowed to cure for three months before being sold. It is stored on the floor of dry caves during

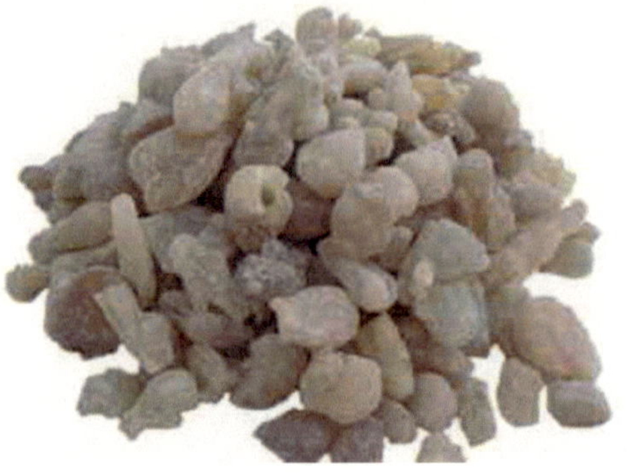

Figure 2. Oleogum Resin Tears of *Boswellia carterii* Birdwood

that period of maturation. The resin occurs in small tears (Fig. 2) varying from 0.5 to 3 cm in length and usually ovoid, pear-shaped, or club-shaped. It is usually of pale yellowish color, frequently with a greenish, bluish or reddish tinge, semi-translucent and covered with a dull white dust, the surface of the tear being dull even after the dust has been removed. They are brittle and internally are opalescent and translucent, the fractured surface being dull and waxy. The drug has a fragrant, balsamic odor and an aromatic, slightly bitter taste, and softens to a plastic mass when chewed. The oleogum resin when triturated with water yields a whitish emulsion (Wallis, 1967).

After such presentation of the deep-rooted usage of frankincense, one can really understand how frankincense is a truly Kings' gift. The oleogum resin of different *Boswellia* species that has various vernacular names *viz.* Frankincense, Incense, or Olibanum in English; Luban Dakar, Bakhor, Kendar in Arabic; Salai guggal In Ayurveda, and H-15 in Germany and Switzerland; was subject to various phytochemical investigations. It is noteworthy that the word Frankincense comes from a 10th century French word meaning "luxuriant incense". The word olibanum is derived from the Hebrew word "Lebonah" and the Greek word "Libanos" meaning white.

The genus takes its name from Professor John Boswell (Miller and Morris, 1988) the uncle of the famous novelist James Boswell, the writer of the well-known Story of Samuel Johnson. The genus comprises several species; all of which are trees (Guenther, 1972 and Lawerence, 1969); of which the most reputed are:

1.2. *Boswellia carterii* Birdwood (Syn. *Boswellia sacra* Flüeckiger)

A tree which is native to Somalia, Southern Yemen (in Hadra'mout valley), and Oman (in Dhofar region). Miller and Morris (Kapoor, 1990) stated that the only species of *Boswellia* present in the Arabian Peninsula is *Boswellia carterii.* This species was named after the English surgeon H.G. Carter who was the first to discover it in his expedition in Southern Arabia at 1846. In 1876, the Swiss chemist and botanist Flüeckiger re-examined the same plant describing it as new species and called it *Boswellia sacra.* Three years later, The English botanist Birdwood reviewed the whole genus and found that the specimens described earlier by Carter and

http://dx.doi.org/10.5772/59006

Flüeckiger are identical to those found in Somalia and Known as *Boswellia carterii* so that the two species should be considered synonymous (Miller and Morris, 1988).

1.3. *Boswellia frereana* Birdwood

A species which is grown in small scale in northern regions of Somalia.

1.4. *Boswellia serrata* Roxb. Ex Colebr.

A species which is grown in India and have been differentiated botanically into two varieties (var. *serrata* with serrated and pubescent leaves, and var. *glabra* with glabrous leaves). Both varieties yield Indian Olibanum.

1.5. *Boswellia papyrifera* (Delile ex Caill.) Hochst

A species which is grown in North Eastern tropical Africa, especially in Sudan (Benson, 1967). The Egyptians supply of the oleogum resin of Frankincense, Olibanum, or Luban dakar comes mainly from Somalia, and rarely from Sudan or Kenya, therefore it is considered to be originated from *Boswellia carterii* Birdwood.

2. Chemistry

A review of the chemistry of Frankincense is made by (Khalid, 1983).

A-The Essential oil:

There has been considerable work done on the composition of olibanum oil from different species and commercial brands of *Boswellia*(Peyron *et al.*, 1980). The volatile oil was found to contain a variety of components *viz.*

Monoterpenes:

In 1978, Obermann investigated the essential oil derived from Aden and Eritrean frankincense and reported that α-pinene is the main component in the Aden oil, whereas n-octyl acetate and n-octanol are the dominant compounds in the Eritrean oil.

In 1978, De Rijke *et al.* isolated traces of the monoterpene acid α-campholytic acid [1] from olibanum oil. This acid was synthesized and showed a rather strong odor reminiscent of the oil. Thus in spite of being a trace constituent, it influences the olfactory character of the oil greatly.

In 1987, Abdel Wahab *et al.* examined the oil of Somali frankincense using GC/MS and found a variety of monoterpene hydrocarbons *viz.* sabinene, camphene, and myrcene; oxides *viz.* cineole; alcohols *viz.* decanol, α-terpineol, and linalol; esters *viz.* bornyl acetate, neryl acetate, and geranyl acetate.

Olibanum oil is reported to contain several odorless cembranoid diterpenes *viz.* cembrene [2], isocembrene [3] (Khalid, 1983) that was initially identified in pine tree resins, whereas

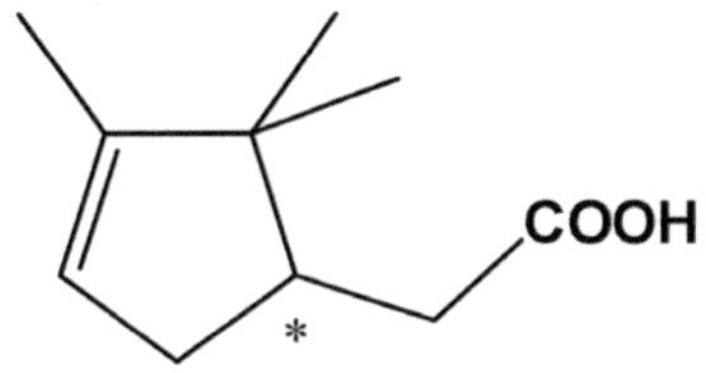

α-campholytic acid

[1]

incensole [4] and the 1-hydroxy derivative [5] occur only in olibanum. These cembranoid macromolecules may in part account for the reported fixative properties of frankincense oil (Ohloff, 1994); just like the macromolecules of Musk oil.

The yield of steam distillation of frankincense essential oil (3%); and its physicochemical constants were determined. Capillary GC/MS technique was used for the analysis of the oil. Several oil components were identified based upon comparison of their mass spectral data with those of reference compounds published in literature or stored in a computer library. The oil was found to contain monoterpenes (13.1 %), sesquiterpenes (1 %), and diterpenes (42.5 %). The chemical profile of the oil is considered as a chemotaxonomical marker that confirmed the botanical and geographical source of the resin (Mikhaeil BR, 2003)

B. The Gum: In 1992, Sen *et al.* were able to isolate and elucidate the structure of 4-O-methyl-glucurono arabinogalactan from the oleogum resin of *Boswellia serrata* Roxb.

C-The Resin:

Several authors reported the isolation and identification of various triterpenes of different skeletons from the resin of different species of the genus *Boswellia*.

2.1. Pentacylic Triterpenes

- Olean-12-ene (β-amyrin type) Triterpenoids:

Classical acid-base extraction procedure led to isolation of α-boswellic acid [58].

In 1972, Elkhadem *et al.* isolated the 3-acetoxy derivative [59] of α-boswellic acid (acetyl α-boswellic acid) by precipitation from ether extract of the resin of the Somaliland variety of olibanum by barium hydroxide followed by acetylation with acetic anhydride and hydrolysis.

Urs-12-ene (α-amyrin type) Triterpenoids: Elkhadem *et al.* were able to eliminate that diene impurity completely by treatment of β-boswellic acid with maleic anydride twice, followed by filtration of the adduct and crystallization. They were able also to prepare different synthetic derivatives of α-, and β-boswellic *viz.* ethyl, ethyl acetyl, and methyl benzoyl esters.

The configurations of such groups and double bond position were later unveiled through progress in NMR spectroscopic techniques especially after 2D-NMR has emerged. Recent advances in crystallographic analysis confirmed the α-configuration of 3-acetoxyl group in

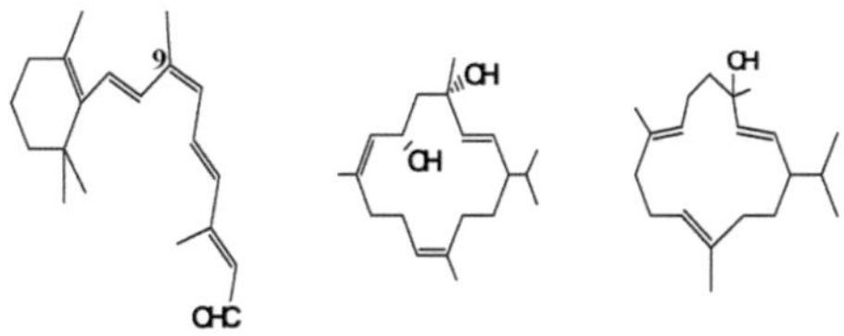

9-cis-retinal [6] | duva-4,8,13-triene-1,3 α-diol [7] | thunbergol [8]

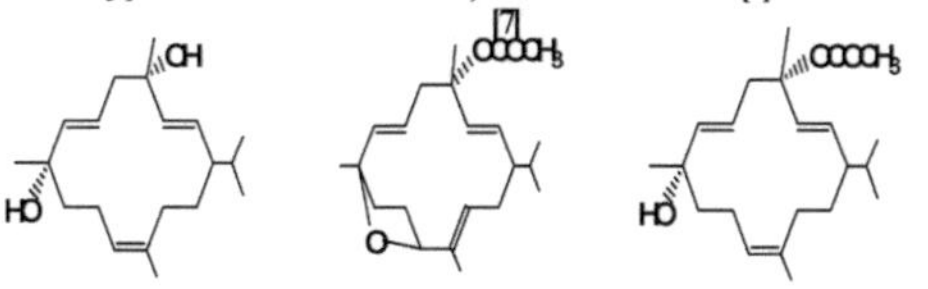

duva-3,9,13-triene-1,5 α-diol [9] | duva-3,9,13-triene-1α-hydroxy-5,8-oxide-1-acetate [10] | duva-3,9,13-triene-1,5α-diol-1-acetate [11]

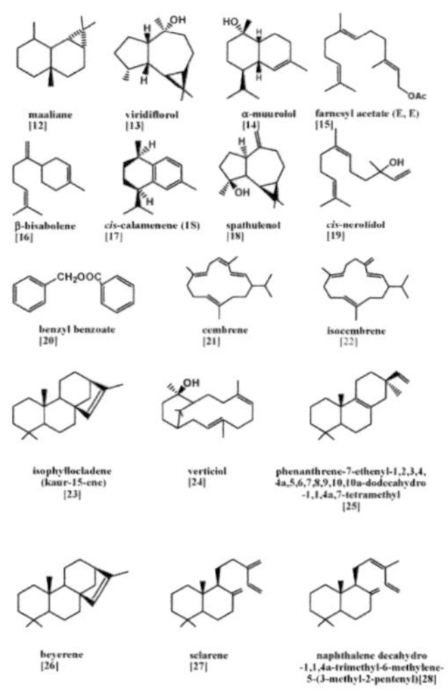

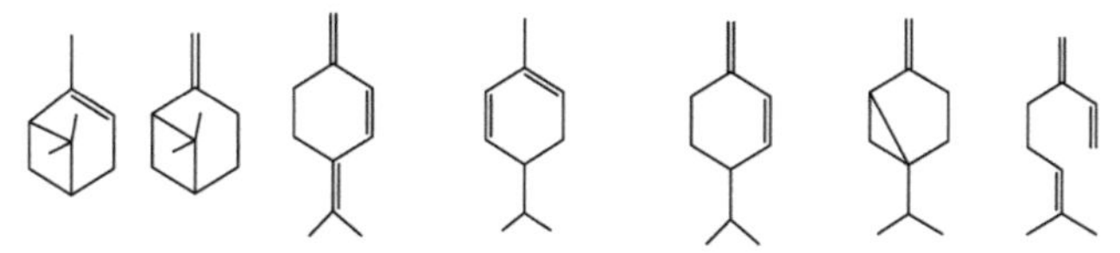

α-pinene [29] | β-pinene [30] | isoterpinolene [31] | α-phellandrene [32] | β-phellandrene [33] | sabinene [34] | β-myrcene [35]

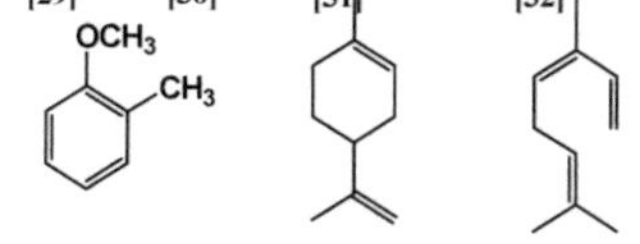

$CH_3—(CH_2)_7—OH$ $CH_3—(CH_2)_7—OCOOH$

o-methyl anisole [36] | *d*-limonene [37] | *cis*-ocimene [38] | octanol [39] | octyl formate [40]

$CH_3—(CH_2)_7OOCCH_3$

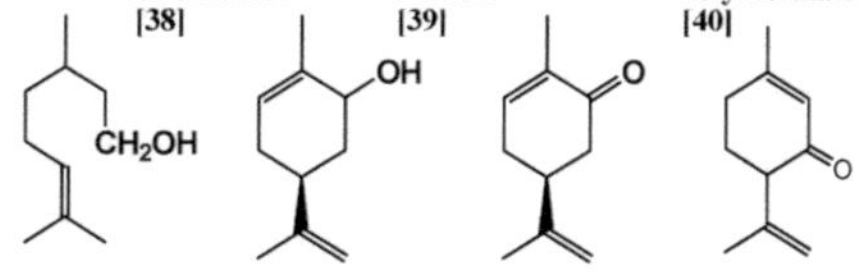

octyl acetate [41] | β-citronellol [42] | *cis*-carveol [43] | carvone [44] | piperitone [45]

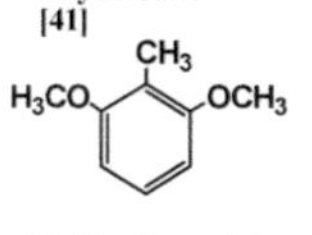

$CH_3(CH_2)_9OH$

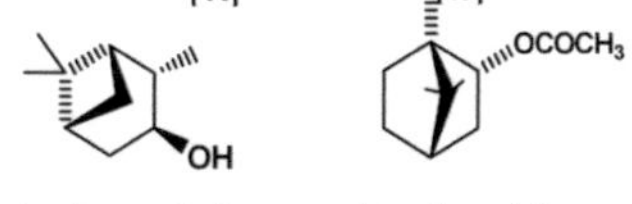

2,6-dimethoxy toluene [46] | 1-decanol [47] | isopinocampheol [48] | bornyl acetate [49]

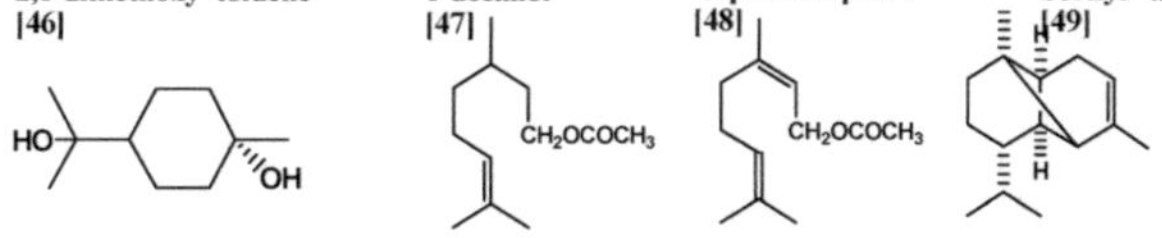

trans-terpin [50] | citronellyl acetate [51] | neryl acetate [52] | α-copaene [53]

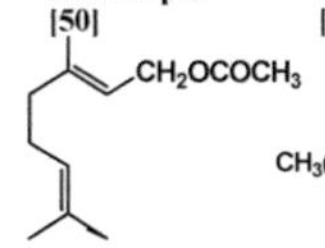

$CH_3(CH_2)_5OCO(CH_2)_4CH_3$ $CH_3(CH_2)_9OCOCH_3$

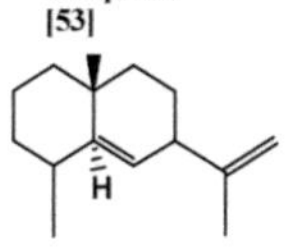

geranyl acetate [54] | hexyl hexanoate [55] | decyl acetate [56] | δ-selinene [57]

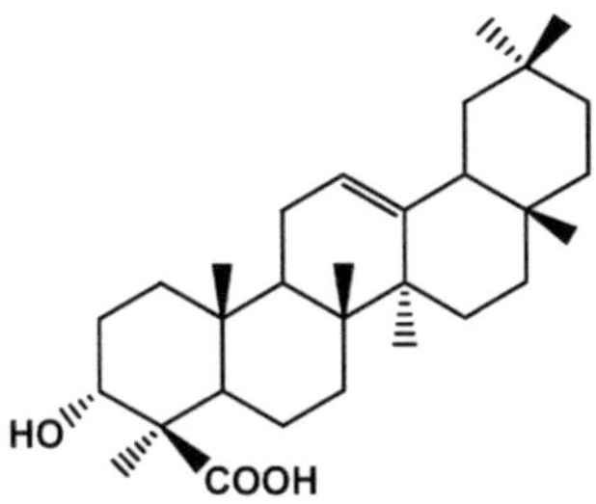

α-Boswellic acid
[58]

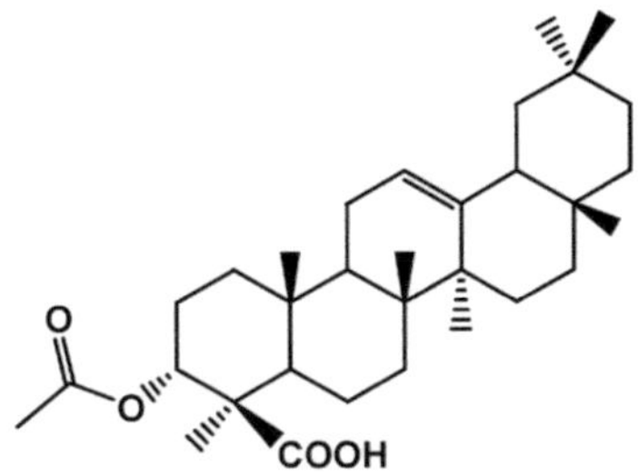

Acetyl-α-Boswellic acid
[59]

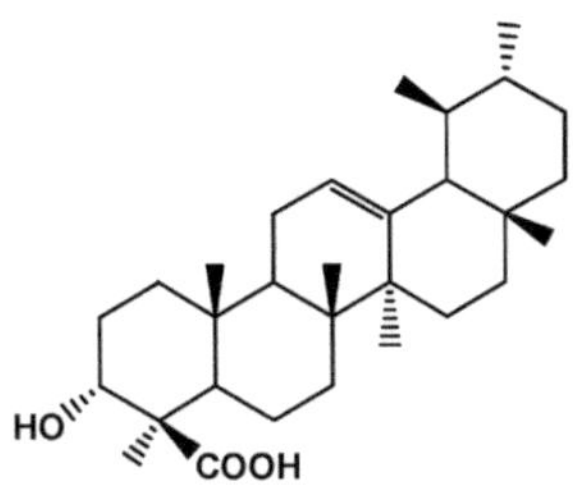

β-Boswellic acid
[60]

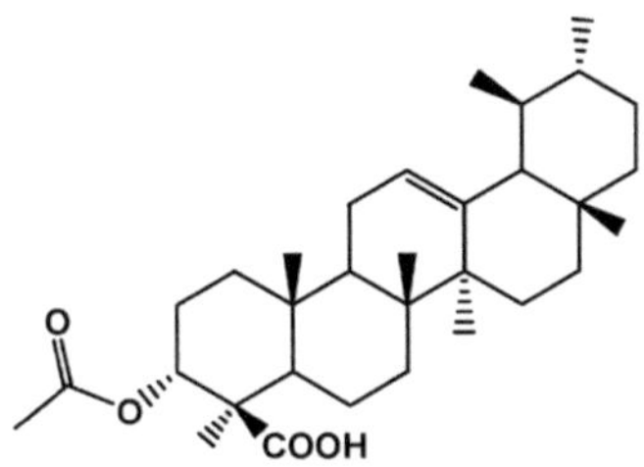

Acetyl β-Boswellic acid
[61]

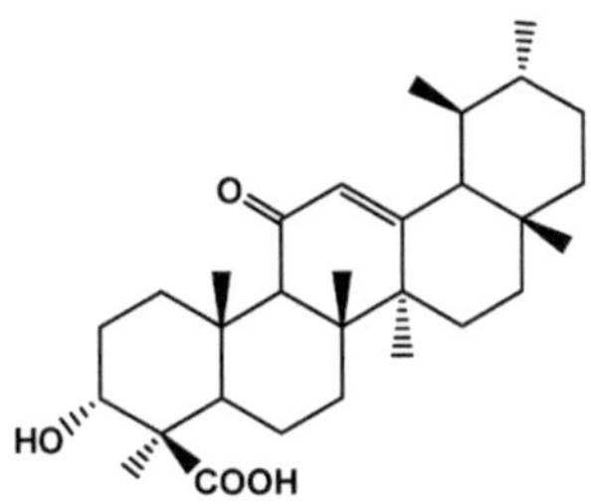

11-Keto -β-Boswellic acid
[62]

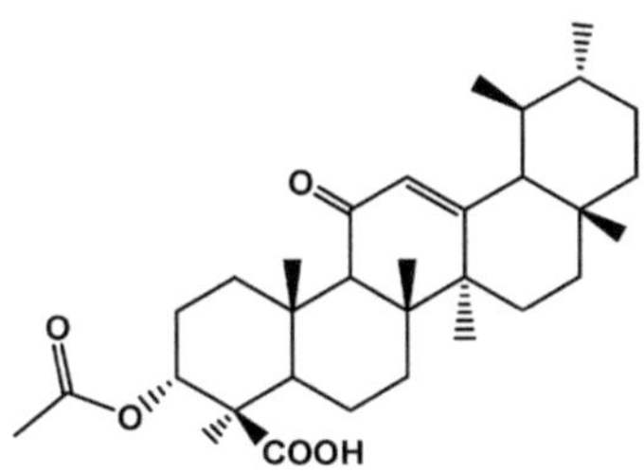

3-O-Acetyl -11-Keto -β-Boswellic acid
[63]

both acetyl-β-boswellic acid, and 3-acetoxyl-11-keto-β-boswellic acid (AKBA) (Schweizer *et* al., 2000).

In 1995, Mahajan *et al.* isolated 3α-hydroxy-urs-9,12-diene-4β-oic acid [64] and 2α, 3α-dihydroxy-urs-12-ene-4-β-oic acid [65] together with other known boswellic acid derivatives by repeated chromatography of the acidic fraction from the ethanolic extract of *Boswellia serrata* Roxb. oleogum resin. They separated also urs-12-ene-3α,24-diol [66] by chromatographic fractionation of the neutral fraction of the resin.

Lupane Triterpenoids:

Proietti *et al.*, 1981 managed to isolate 2 lupane-skeleton triterpenoids from resin exudate of *Boswellia frereana* distributed in the northern regions of Somalia namely, lupeol [67] and epilupeol [68].

http://dx.doi.org/10.5772/59006

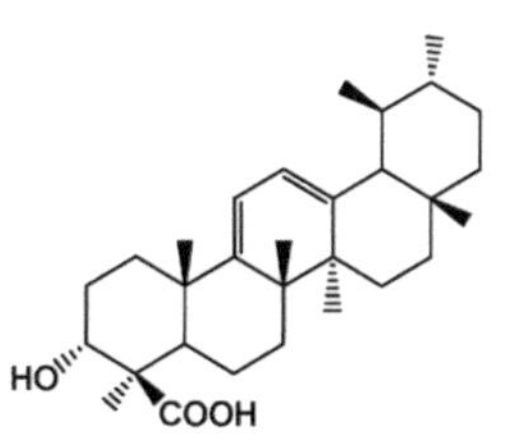

(3α-Hydroxy-urs-9,12-diene-4-β-oic acid)
[64]

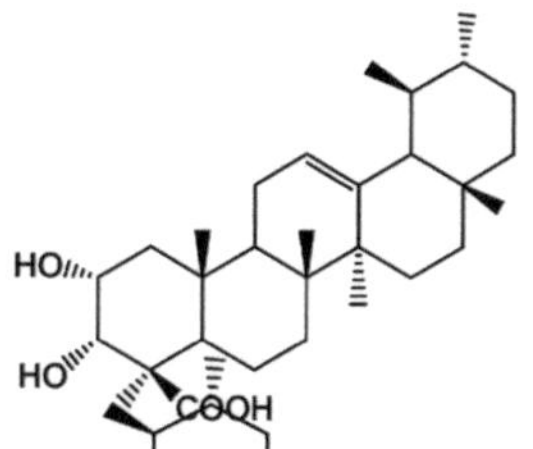

(2α,3α-dihydroxy -urs-12-ene-4-β-oic acid)
[65]

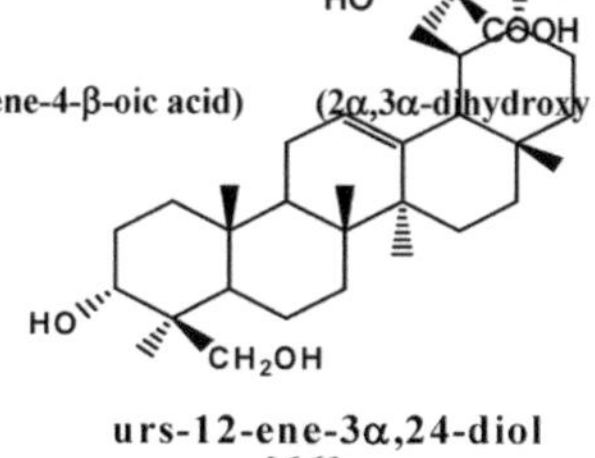

urs-12-ene-3α,24-diol
[66]

2.2. Tetracyclic triterpenes

Tirucallane Triterpenoids:

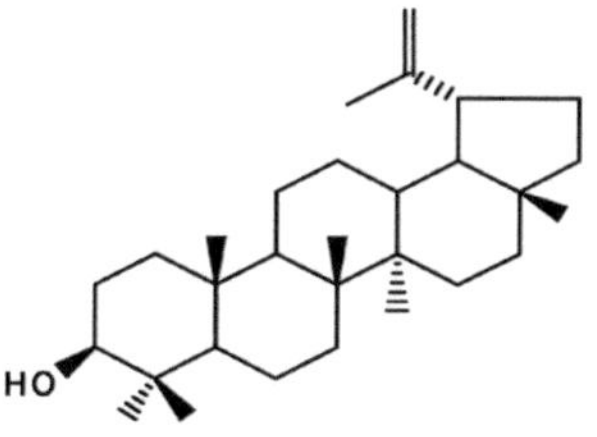

Lupeol
[67]

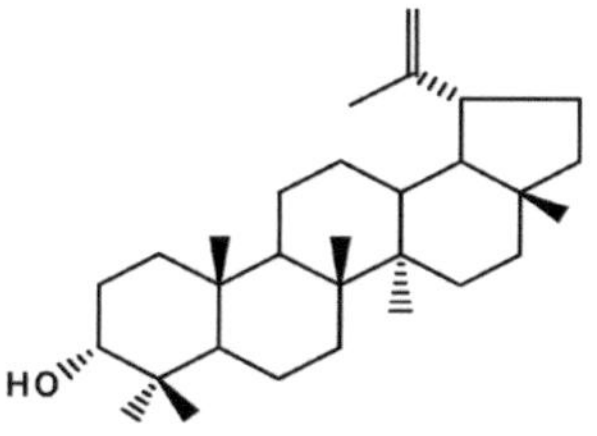

Epilupeol
[68]

Liang *et al.*, (22) reported the presence of a variety of tirucallane triterpenoids in family Burseraceae.

In 2001, Boden *et al.* reported isolation of three triterpenoids having tirucallane nucleus from the oleogum resin of *Boswellia serrata* Roxb. ; namely 3-keto-8,24-diene-21-β-oic acid (3-oxo-tirucallic acid) [69], 3-β-hydroxy-tirucall-8,24-diene-21-β-oic acid (3-hydroxy-tirucallic acid) [70], and 3-β-acetoxy-tirucall-8,24-diene-21-β-oic acid (3-acetoxy- tirucallic acid) [71].

Dammarane triterpenoids:

In 1985, Fattorusso *et al.* isolated four dammarane triterpenes from the most polar fractions of the chloroformic extract of the exudate of *Boswellia frereana*, namely 3β-acetoxy-16(S),20(R)-dihydroxy dammar-24-ene [72], 3β,20(S)-dihydroxy dammar-24-ene [73], its 3-acetyl derivative [74], and 20(S)-protopanaxdiol [75].

- 3,4- Secotriterpenoids:

3,4-secotriterpenic acids carrying an isopropyl group at position 5 are very rare as naturally occurring compounds. They are considered to be degradation products originating through

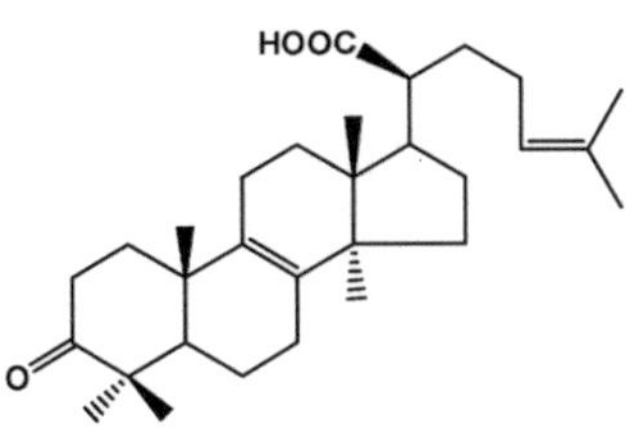

(3-oxo tirucallic acid)
[69]

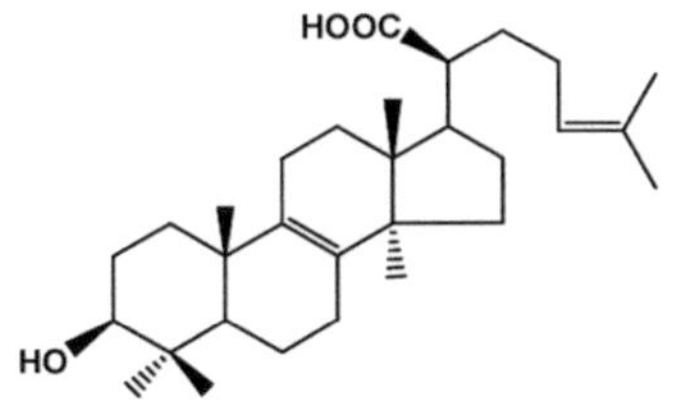

(3β-Hydroxy tirucallic acid)
[70]

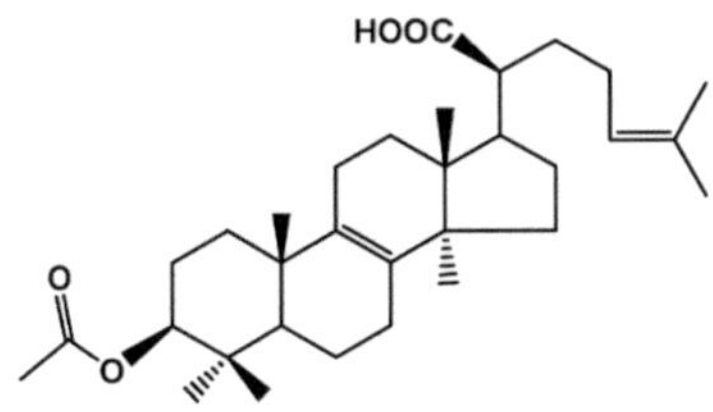

(3β-Acetoxy tirucallic acid)
[71]

geochemical process involving photochemical or photomimetic reactions. In 1983, Fattorusso *et al.* managed to isolate a member of such group of compounds, namely 4(23)-dihydro roburic acid [76] from the acidic fraction of incense *Boswellia carterii* Birdwood after methylation with diazomethane followed by catalytic hydrogenation of the produced methyl ester and column chromatography.

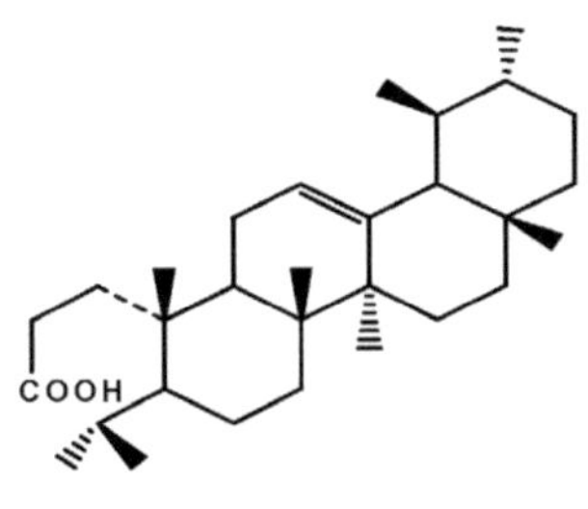

4(23)-Dihydro roburic acid
[76]

Analysis of the oleogum resin:

In 2001, Ganzera and Khan developed a reversed phase HPLC method for the separation of boswellic acids from *Boswellia serrata* oleogum resin. The first accurate determination of 6 individual acids was possible in the resin as well as in multi-component preparations. By using an acidic mobile phase, raised temperature, and a 4 μm Synergi MAX-RP 80 A column, the acids could be detected at levels as low as 0.9 μg/ml. The study of market products revealed significant variations in the content of these pharmacologically active compounds in commercial samples. (Ganzera & Khan, 2001)

Assignment of other atoms was made by referring to reported compilation data of a variety of similar compounds (Mahato *et al.*, 1994), and by using data from DEPT spectrum combined with ^{1}H-^{1}H COSY, HMQC correlations and long range C-H correlation data from HMBC spectrum which is illustrated by (Fig. 3). EI/MS fragments corroborated the aforementioned assignments showing a molecular ion peak $[M]^{+}$ at m/z 512.35 corresponding for the molecular formula $C_{32}H_{48}O_{5}$.

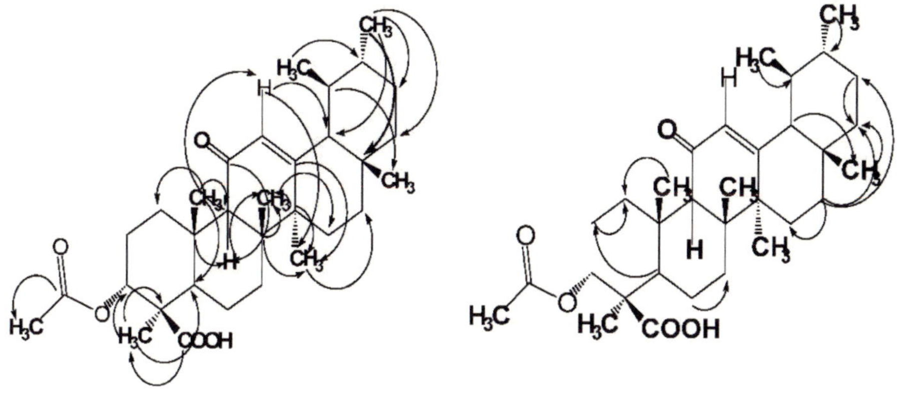

Figure 3. HMBC Correlation for 3-acetyl 11-keto β-Boswellic acid [63]

From the above mentioned data, and from literature data; one can conclude that compound A-6 is 3α-acetoxy-urs-12-ene-11-Keto-24β-oic acid known as acetyl-11-Keto-β-Boswellic acid (AKBA). A computer- generated model for that compound after energy minimization using

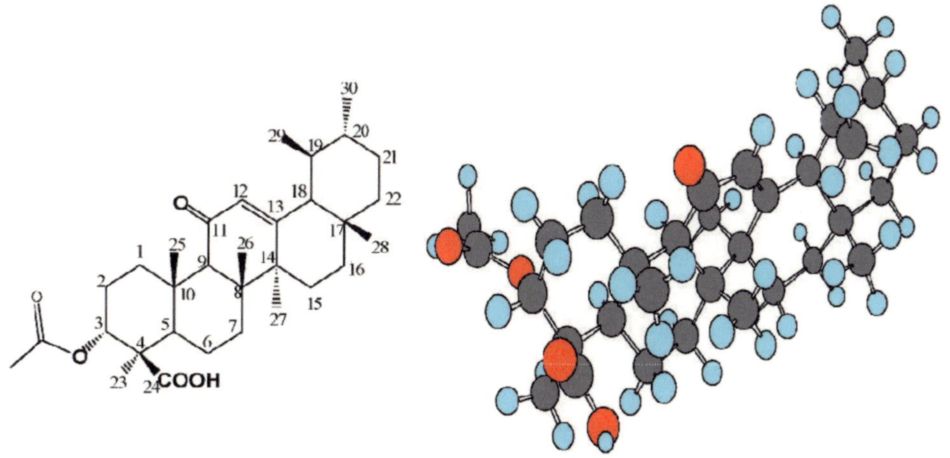

Figure 4. Computer-generated Model of 3-acetyl 11-keto β-Boswellic acid [63]

CSChem3D program pro-version 4.0 (Cambridge Soft Corp.) is shown in Fig. 4.

The aforementioned data; it was suggested that 3α-hydroxy-urs-12-ene-11-keto-24β-oic acid known as 11-keto β-Boswellic acid (Kβ-BA). A computer-generated model for that compound after energy minimization using CSChem3D program pro-version 4.0 (Cambridge Soft Corp.) is shown in (Fig. 5).

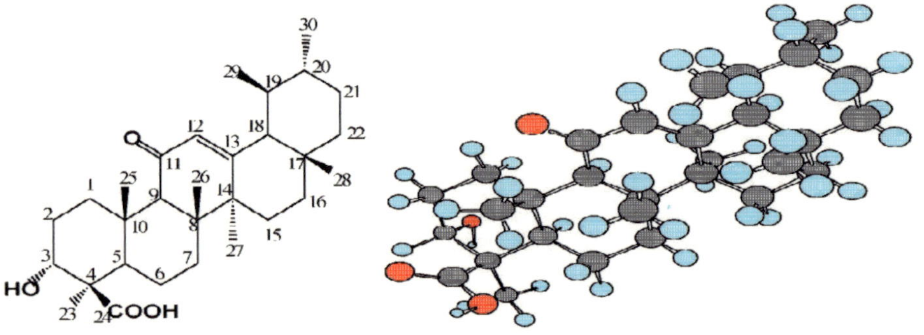

Figure 5. Computer-generated Model of 11-Keto-β-Boswellic acid [62]

3. Biology

- Rough based Granular computing approach had been used to predict response to new medication from Boswellia and other components for treatment of HCV patients as presented in Fig. 6 (Badria et. Al al. 2013).

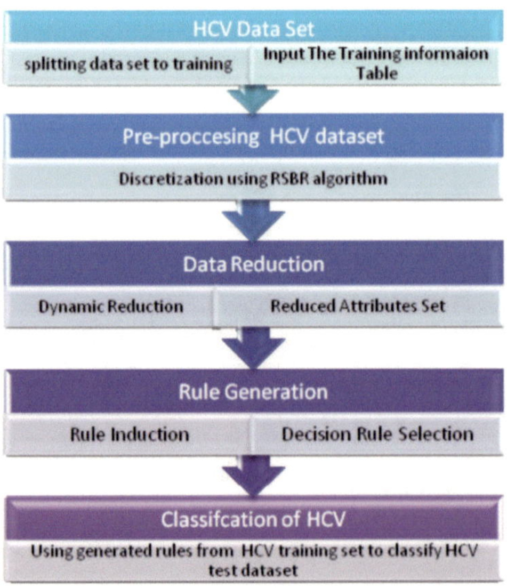

Figure 6. Rough based Granular Approach (RGA) Used in HCV Dataset Classification

http://dx.doi.org/10.5772/59006

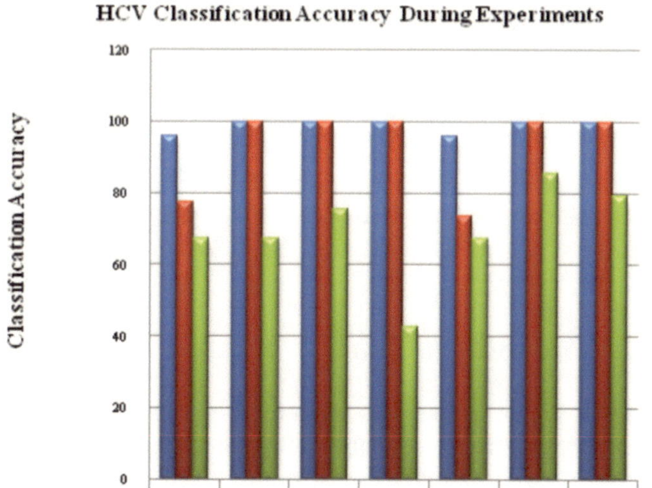

	R1	R2	R3	R4	R5	R6	R7
3 Months	95.9	100	100	100	95.9	100	100
6 Months	77.6	100	100	100	73.5	100	100
9 Months	67.3	67.3	75.5	42.8	67.3	85.7	79.5

Figure 7. Classifications Accuracy for Each Reduct During Experiment

- *Boswellia carterii* extract in combination with glycyrrhizin (Badria *et al.* 2003) showed a strong biochemical and histopathological hepatoprotective effect on rat Liver Injury.
- Frankincense triterpenoids showed Anti-Herpes activity (Badria *et al.* 2003) and Immunomodulatory effects (Badria *et al.* 2003 and Botros *et al.* 2003).
- Animal studies showed that the ingestion of a defatted alcoholic extract of *Boswellia* decreased polymorphonuclear leukocyte infiltration and migration, decreased primary antibody synthesis (Sharma and Singh, 1989) and caused almost total inhibition of the classical complement pathway (Wagner, 1989) and alternate complement system (Knaus and Wagner, 1996).
- The gum resin extract from *Boswellia was* recently shown to have positive therapeutic effects in inflammatory bowel disease. However, the mechanisms and constituents responsible for these effects are poorly understood (Krielgstein, 2001). Moreover, in a clinical study reported that *Boswellia* extract appears to be superior over mesalazine in terms of a benefit-risk-evaluation (Gehardt *et al.*, 2001).
- β-boswellic acid and its derivatives have anti-tumor and antihyperlipidemic activities (Huan et al., 2000).
- *Boswellia* has also been observed to inhibit human leukocyte elastase (Safayhi *et al.*, 1997 and Schweizer *et al.*, 2000): Boswellic acids are effective anti-inflammatory and anti-arthritis agents,they also help control high blood lipids and protect the liver against bacterial

galactosamine -endotoxin. The non acid part of the gum has pain relieving and sedative qualities, and in high doses can lower blood pressure, and reduce heart rate in dogs but increase in frogs observed benefits of *Boswellia* include reduction in joint swelling, increased mobility, steroid sparing action, less morning stiffness, improved grip strength, and general improvement in quality of life, for both osteoarthritis and rheumatoid arthritis. (Pachnanda et al. 1996).

- Boswellia gum has been used for the treatment of diabetes, skin and blood diseases, fever, cardiovascular disorders, neurological disorders, dysentery and diseases of the tests (Adrian, 1998).

3.1. Predicting the Effect of Boswellic Acid

If the boswellic acid was just another leukotriene inhibitor, then its effects probably could be predicted on the basis of these drugs: It probably works sometimes, it probably doesn't work for everyone, it probably is very effective for aspirin-induced asthma, it isn't going to be quite as strong as corticosteroids, and it isn't going to have as big an effect on the amount of air that can be expelled in one second as it does on other symptoms. These are, in fact, reasonable expectations (Safahyi *et al.*, 1992). However, the boswellic acids neutralize elastase (Safahyi *et al.*, 1997). It is not known how important this is. First, it is not known to what extent elastase contributes to the problem of asthma. Second, it is not known to what extent elastase is a problem when taking a leukotriene inhibitor (Safahyi *et al.*, 1997). Boswellic acid's ability to neutralize elastase is superfluous, or it might nicely complement the inhibition of leukotrienes. Also, we don't know how much the boswellic acids actually neutralize elastase.

3.2. Experimental Autoimmune Encephalomyelitis (Multiple Sclerosis)

Wildfeuer et al., 1998 administered a mixture of acetyl-boswellic acids to guinea pigs with experimental autoimmune encephalomyelitis. Multiple sclerosis occurs when the myelin insulating the neurons in the brain is destroyed. Researchers wishing to study this can't wait for rats to get multiple sclerosis. Instead, they create a problem that is much like multiple sclerosis, which is called experimental autoimmune encephalomyelitis (Wildfeuer et al., 1998). Two studies (Safayhi *et al.*, 1992) had previously found that leukotriene inhibitors reduced the development of experimental autoimmune encephalomyelitis. Of course, there is a jump from experimental autoimmune encephalomyelitis in a rodent to multiple sclerosis in a human. Curiously, the role of leukotrienes in multiple sclerosis seems to have garnered more attention. People with multiple sclerosis do have increased leukotrienes (Sailer *et al.* 1996).

4. Blocking the formation of leukotrienes

4.1. Leukotrienes Inhibitors

Safahyi *et al.*, 1992, observed the ability of the different boswellic acids to inhibit the formation of the leukotriene LTB4. As noted, the other leukotrienes are more important with regard to asthma. However, the mode of action of the boswellic acids should be equally effective for all leukotrienes, because they inhibit 5-lipoxygenase, the key enzyme needed for starting the synthesis of all leukotrienes. Safahyi and his group (1992) measured the concentration needed to block the activity of LTB4 by 50%. For AKBA, the needed concentration was 1.5 micromoles.

For the other boswellic acids, it was 4-7 micromoles, which means that 3 to 4 times greater a concentration was needed. A factor of 3 or 4 might not be that important as things go, but this finding singled out AKBA as being the most powerful boswellic acids (Safahyi *et al.*, 1992). Wildfeuer et al., 1998, found that boswellic acids reduce leukotriene formation, and AKBA is the most effective.

5. Clinical applications

5.1. For treatment of knee osteoarthritis

After one month of treatment there was a significant reduction of pain on active movement, passive movement, tenderness, nocturnal pain and a significant improvement of pain free walking time. After two months of therapy, there was a highly significant reduction of pain on active movement, pain on passive movement, tenderness, nocturnal pain, and highly significant prolongation of pain free walking time. At the end of three months, there was a significant reduction of grade of knee effusion, with highly significant reduction of pain on passive movement, pain on active movement, tenderness, and significant prolongation of pain free walking time (Badria *et al.* 2004).

Efficacy and tolerability of *Boswellia* and turmeric in this work is superior to clinical trial of NSAIDs in treatment of active osteoarthritis. The efficacy of NSAIDs (diclofenace) were tested in a double blind clinical trail in 50 OA patients at dose of 50 mg bid for three weeks and follow up visit after seven weeks. At the end of the trial, there was a significant reduction in pain, joint tenderness ($P < 0.05$) and swelling (Badria *et al.* 2002).

5.2. For treatment of bronchial asthma

Badria *et. al, 2002* and Gupta *et al,* 1998 performed the best type of research study in a double-blind, placebo-controlled study. Some subjects with bronchial asthma. During the 6 week treatment period, the subjects taking boswellic acid had an average of.3 asthmatic attacks and the subjects taking the placebo had an average of 1.2. despite worse starting signs, the subjects taking boswellic acid actually had fewer asthmatic attacks. Therefore, Gupta's study stands as good evidence that boswellic acid at least reduces the probability of an asthmatic attack (Gupta *et al,* 1998).

After 2 weeks treatment with boswellia, there was a significant increase in both FEV1 and PEFR ($P \leq 0.05$ and ≤ 0.01 respectively) with no significant change in FVC in the severe persistent asthma subgroup (C1) when compared to those received placebo (C2). The potent inhibitory action of boswellia extract on blood eosinophils, can be explained by a potent anti-inflammatory action extends beyond the leukotriene inhibition (Badria et al. 2004).

5.2.1. Ulcerative colitis

Badria *et al.,* 2001 and Gupta *et. al.* 1997 compared boswellic acid to a typical therapy for ulcerative colitis, sulfasalazine. To roughly characterize the finding, there was no observable difference between the two treatments (Badria *et al.,* 2001)

5.3. For treatment of hepatitis C

Inclusion Criteria:

- positive PCR for HCV.
- Elevated liver enzymes within 6 months of the Entry, with no attribution to causes other than HCV
- Chronic HCV confirmed histologically with Liver biopsy within 2 years of entry
- Both genders were eligible within age of 18-70 years old.

Participants were enlisted from a group of HCV-infected patients currently enrolled in a large observational study in Egypt. Participants received the supplements daily for 18 months, with measures obtained every 6 months.

Measures to be assessed will include: compliance with assignment, retention in the study, Liver enzymes levels, serum collagen markers, self-described symptoms, viral load and clearance, abdominal ultrasound. It is hypothesized that the supplements led to clearance of HCV infections and/or at least prevent progression of liver disease in participants with chronic HCV hepatitis and, in some cases, reverse hepatic lesions that are already present, as well as improving the quality of life in individuals who use this dietary supplement. (Badria *et al.* 2002)

Author details

Farid A. Badria*

Address all correspondence to: faridbadria@yahoo.com

Pharmacognosy Department, Faculty of Pharmacy, Mansoura University, Mansoura, Egypt

References

[1] Abdel wahab S. M., Aboutabl E. A., Elzalabani S. M., Fouad H. A., De Pooter H. L., and El Fallaha B.; (1987), The Essential Oil of Olibanum, *Planta Medica*, 53, 382.

[2] Adrian AL(1996), Boswellia serrata. A unique Ayuvredic Anti-rheumatic. Issue of VRP's Nutritional News.

[3] Badria F., Mohammed E., El-Badrawy M., and El-Desouky M., (2004), Natural Leukotriene Inhibitor from Boswellia: A Potential New Alternative for Treating Bronchial Asthma, Alternative Complementary Therapies; 10(5), 257-265.

[4] Badria F., El-Farahaty, Shabana A., Hawas S., and El-Batoty M.F., (2002), Boswellia-Curcumin Preparation for Treating Knee Osteoarthritis: A Clinical Evaluation,. Altern. Complement. Ther.; 8(6), 341-8.

[5] Badria, F.(2001), Method Of Preparation A New Pharmaceutical product composed of Curcumin, Glycyrrhizin, and Acid extract of Boswellia Carterii Based upon induction of Endogenous Interferon, Egyptian Patent # 23375, (December 2, 2002 to December 1, 2022), Egypt.

[6] Badria, F.(2001), Preparation a new product of Natural origin for treatment of hyperacidity and colitis, Egyptian Patent # 23376. (April 30, 2001 expires April 29, 2021,Egypt).

[7] Badria, Farid A., Houssen, Wael E., El-Nashar, Eman M. and Saaed, Sheheta A, (2003), Effect of Glycyrrhizin and *Boswellia carterii* extract on Liver Injury: Biochemical and Histopathological Evaluation, Biosci. Biotech. Res. Asia; 1(2), 93-96.

[8] Badria, Farid A., Mohamed Abu-Karam, Botros R. Mikhaeil, Galal T. Maatooq, and Mohamed M. Amer, (2003), Anti-Herpes Activity of Isolated Compounds from Frankincense, Biosci. Biotech. Res. Asia.; 1(1), 1-10.

[9] Badria, Farid A., Botros R. Mikhaeil, Galal T. Maatooq, and Mohamed M. Amer; (2003), Immunomodulatory Triterpenoids from Frankincense, Z. Naturforschung,; 58c 505-516.

[10] Badria, Farid A., Eissa, Mohammed M., Elmogy, Mohammed., Hashem, Mohammed, (2013), Rough Based Granular Computing Approach for Making Treatment Decisions of Hepatitis C, ICCTA, 29-31 October 2013, Alexandria, Egypt

[11] Benson L.; (1976), *"Plant Classification"*, 2nd Indian reprint, Oxford & IBH Publishing Co., New Delhi, p.170.

[12] Boden S. E., Schweizer S., Bertsche T., Dufer M., Drews G., and Safayhi H.; (2001) *Molecular Pharmacology*, 60, 267.

[13] Botros R. Mikhaeil, Galal T. Maatooq, Farid A. Badria and Mohammed M. Amer.; (2003), Chemistry and immunomodulatory Activity of Frankincense oil Z. Naturforschung, 58c, 230-238

[14] Chopra R. N., Nayer S. L., and Chopra I. C.; (1956), *"Glossary of Indian Medicinal Plants"*, Council of scientific and Industrial Research, New Delhi.

[15] D.de Rijke, P. C. Traas, R. ter Heide, H. Boelens and H. J. Takken, (1978), Acidic components in essential oils of costus root, patchouli and olibanum *Phytochemistry*, 17(9), 1664-1666.

[16] El-Khadem H., El-Shafei Z. M., El-Sekeily M. A. S., and Abdel Rahman M. M. A.; (1972), *Planta Medica*, 22, 157.

[17] Fattorusso E., Santacroce C., and Xaasan C.F.; (1983), 4(23)-Dihydroroburic acid from the Resin (Incense) of *Boswellia Carterii*, Phytochemistry, 22, 2868.

[18] Fattorusso E., Santacroce C., and Xaasan C.F.; (1985), Dammarane Triterpenes from the Resin of *Boswellia freerana*, Phytochemistry; 24, 1035.

[19] Ganzera M., and Khan I. A.; (2001), A Reversed Phase High Performance Liquid Chromatography Method for the Analysis of Boswellic acids in *Boswellia serrata*, Planta *Medica*, 67, 778.

[20] Gerhardt H, Seifert F, Buvari P, Vogelsang H, Repges R, (2001), Therapy of active Crohn disease with Boswellia serrata extract H15Z. Gastroenterol; 39(1): 11-7.

[21] Guenther E.; (1972), "*The Essential Oils*", Vol. IV, Robert E. Krieger Publishing Co., Huntington, New York; pp. 352-356.

[22] Gupta I, Gupta V, Parihar A, Gupta S, Ludtke R, Safayhi, Ammon HP(1998): Effects of Boswellia serrata gum resin in patients with bronchial asthma. Eur J Med Resp; 3(11): 511-4.

[23] Gupta I, Parihar A, Malhorta P(1997), : Effects of *Boswellia serrata* gum resin in patients with ulcerative colitis. Eur J Med Res; 2: 37: 4

[24] Huan MT, Badmaev V, Ding Y, Liu Y, Xie JG, Ho CT, (2000), Antitumor and anticarcinogenic activities of triter period, beta-boswellic acid. In Biofactors; 13(1-4): 225-30.

[25] Kapoor L. D.; (1990), "*CRC Handbook of Ayurvedic Medicinal Plants*", CRC Press, Florida, USA, p. 83.

[26] Khalid S. A.; (1983), "*Chemistry of the Burseraceae*", Annual Proceedings Phytochemical, Society of Europe, 22, 281-299.

[27] Knaus U, Wagner H, (1996), Effects of boswellic acid of Boswellia serrata and other triterpenic acids on the complement system. Phytomedicine; 3: 77-81.

[28] Krieglstein CF, Anthoni C, Rijcken EJ, Laukotter M, Spiegel HU, Boden SE, Schweizer S, Safayhi H, Senninger N and Schurmann G, (2001), Acetyl-11-Keto-beta-boswellic acid, a constituent of a herbal medicine from Boswellia serrata resin, attenuates experimental ileitis. Int J Colorectal Dis; 16(2):88-95.

[29] Lawrence G. H.; (1969), "*Taxonomy of Vascular Plants*"; 2nd Indian reprint, Oxford & IBH Publishing Co., Calcutta, India, p. 559.

[30] Liang G. Y., Gray A. I., Waterman P. G.;. (1988), Tirucallane and Oleanane Triterpenes from the Resin of Aucoumea Klaineana, *Phytochemistry*, 27, 2283.

[31] Mahajan B., Taneja S. C., Sethi V. K., and Dhar K. L.; (1995), Two Triterpenoids from *Boswellia serrata* gum resin, *Phytochemistry*, 39, 453-5.

[32] Mahato, S. B., and Kundu A. P.; (1994), ^{13}C-NMR Spectra of Pentacyclic Triterpenoids-A Compilation and Some Salient Features, Phytochemistry, 37, 1517.

[33] Mikhaeil BR, Maatooq GT, Badria FA, Amer MM.; (2003), "Chemistry and immunomodulatory activity of frankincense oil.", Z Naturforsch C. 58, 230-8.

[34] Miller A. G., and Morris M.; (1988), "*Plants of Dhofar, The Southern Region of Oman. Traditional, Economic and Medicinal uses*", The Office of the Advisor for Conservation of the Environment, Diwan of Royal Court, Sultanate of Oman, pp. 78-81

[35] Murray T. M.; (1995), "*The Healing power of Herbs*", Prima publishing.

[36] Singh G. B., and Atal C. K. (1986), Pharmacology of an extract of Salai guggal ex-*Boswellia serrata*, a new non-steroidal anti-inflammatory agent. Agents Actions 18, 407-412.

[37] Obermann H. (1978), Monoterpensäuren als Spurenkomonenten in Olibanumöl. *Dragoco Rep.* 3, 55-58.

[38] Ohloff G.; (1994), "*Scent and fragrances*"; Translated by Pickenhagen W., and Lawrence B. M., Springer-Verlag, Berlin, Heidelberg, 187.

[39] Pachnanda et al. ; (1996), The Wealth of Asia, Ind. J. Pharmacol., 1981;13: 63.

[40] Peyron L., Accchiardi J., Bignotti D., and Pellerin P.; (1980, October), *International Congress of Essential Oils*, Cannes, P. 95.

[41] Proietti G., Strappaghetti G., and Corsano S.; (1981), *Planta Medica*, 4, 417.

[42] Ryman D.; (1997), "*Aromatherapy*", Judy Piatkus Publishers Ltd., London, pp. 101-102.

[43] Schweizer S, Von Brocke AF, Boden SE, Bayer E, Ammon HP and Safayhi H, (2000), Work-up dependent formation of 5-lipoxygenase-inhibitory boswellic acid analogues J Nat Prod; 63: 1058-61.

[44] Safayhi H., Mack T., Sabieraj J., Anazodo M. I., Subramanian L. R. and Ammon H. P. T.; (1992), *Journal of Pharmacology and Experimental Therapeutics*, 261, 1143.

[45] Safayhi H, Rall B, Sailer ER, Ammon HPT, (1997) Inhibition by Boswellic acids of human leukocyte elastase. J Pharmacol Exp Ther; 281: 460-463.

[46] Sailer E. R., Subramanian L. R., Rall B., Hoernlein R. F., Ammon H. P. T., and Safayhi H.; (1996), *British Journal of Pharmacology*, 117, 615.

[47] Sen A. K., Das A. K., Banerji N., Vignon M. R., (1992), Isolation and structure of a 4-O-methyl-glucouroarabinogalactan from Boswellia serrata, Carbohy. Res. 223, 321-7.

[48] Sharma ML, Bani S, Singh GB; (1989), Antiarthritic activity of boswellic acid in bovine serum albumin-induced arthritis. In J Immunopharm; 6:647-652.

[49] Wagner H: (19899, Search for new plant constituents with potential antiphlogistic and antiallergic activity. Planta Medica; 55:235-241.

[50] Wallis T. E.; (1967), "*Text book of Pharmacognosy*", 5th Ed., J. & A. Churchill Ltd., pp. 500-501.

[51] Wildfeuer A., Neu I. S., Safayhi H., Metzger G., Wehrmann M., Vogel U., and Ammon H. P. (1998), T.; *Arzneimittel Forschung/Drug research*, 48, 668.

Chapter 2

Evaluation of *Glycyrrhiza glabra* Cream as Treatment for Melasma

Amina Hamed Alobaidi, Eqbal Salih Hamad,
Abdulghani Mohamed Alsamarai and
Kudair Abass Kudair

Additional information is available at the end of the chapter

http://dx.doi.org/10.5772/58918

1. Introduction

Melasma is a common cosmetic problem in our community [1], with social and psychological burden. It is a disorder of pigmentary system characterized by irregular brown or grayish-brown, acquired hypermelanosis of sun-exposed areas especially the face [2]. Many preparations were used for treatment of melasma, but none of them was ideal [3].

Researchers recently are more involved in performing a research that evaluated the therapeutic effects of formulation that with active substance of plant origin [4]

Recently, topical polyherbal formulations are the latest additions to the treatment approaches list of melasma, with a reducing and diverting the production of melanin [5]. The therapeutic effect of such preparation was enhanced when cosmetic emulsion contained antioxidants are used as active ingredients [6]. Natural herbs are a rich source of many antioxidatively acting compounds [7]. *Glycyrrhiza glabra* is a medicinal plant with rich natural antioxidants [8].The best natural antioxidants in extract of *Glycyrrhiza glabra* are glycyrrhizin (glycyrrhizic acid) and flavonoids [9]. The role of plant extract of *Glycyrrhiza glabra* on skin is mainly attributed to its antioxidant activity particularly to its potent antioxidants triterpene, saponins and flavonoids [10]. G. glabra extract are with therapeutic effects in skin whitening [11], skin depigmenting [12], skin lightening [3], antiaging [14], anti-erythemic [14], emollient [15], anti-acne [16] and photoprotection effects [17,18]. A 2.5% G. glabra extract cream was formulated and it was with sound chemical and physical stability [19]. In this study, 2.5% of G. glabra extract was evaluated as treatment of melasma in female.

2. Materials and methods

2.1. Study design

Double blind placebo controlled study. The study population stratified to active or placebo treatment randomly. The female with even code number receiving cream with active ingredient while female with odd code number receiving placebo. The cream distributed by a pharmacist, while the clinical evaluation was performed by a dermatologist clinician.

2.2. Study population

Hundred female volunteers were enrolled in this study between the ages of 20 and 45 years. They were recruited from Dermatology Clinic in Samarra Teaching Hospital and daily dermatology clinics. Prior to the tests, the volunteers were examined for any serious skin disease or damage especially on cheeks and forearms. Before the study, every volunteer was provided with a volunteer protocol. This protocol stating the terms and conditions of the testing were to be signed by every volunteer individually. Blood samples were collected from the 100 volunteer females suffering from melasma.They were diagnosed by consultant dermatologists. Wood's lamp (340-400) nm was used to identify the types of melasma whether epidermal, dermal or mixed (dermoepidermal). Of the total 76%were married and 24% were single. Serum of the patients and controls were investigated for levels of TSH, estrogen, progesterone, prolactin, ALT (SGPT), AST (SGOT), total protein, blood urea and S. albumin before and after treatment.

The history as well as personal information about patients was obtained by questionnaire. Volunteers were not informed about the contents of formulations. All the skin tests have been done at 25°C. Erythema of the skin are determined on the first day before application of any cream and then on days 7, 14, 21 and 28 after treatment. Fifty female from patients group received the treatment for 28 days, 7 patients were lost to follow up. The above parameters for forty three patients were determined after treatment. As well as fifty female suffering from melasma took the placebo, the same above parameters were measured before and after treatment.

None of the patients or control subjects was on any oral and/or local medication. The pregnant and lactating females or patients on any hormonal therapy (contraceptive pills) were excluded from the study. Patients with other systemic diseases like diabetes, hypertension, or on drugs for any underlying disease were also excluded.

2.3. Formulation

Water in oil (W/O) active cream (2.5% G. glabra) and base were prepared as described previously [19].

3. Results

3.1. Age and marital status

A 100 female suffering from melasma, 93 completed the study while 7 patients were lost to follow up. The distribution of these two groups is shown in Table (1). They were divided into 3 age groups. The highest percentages (50%) and (56%) were found in the age group of (30-39) years for active cream and control patient groups respectively. The lowest percentage of incidence for active treatment females was (12%) in the age group of (40-50) years, and for control, the lowest percentage was (4%) in the age group of (40-50) years. The highest incidence of melasma was found in married women than in singles of both groups, Table (1).

	Formulation			Placebo		
Age group	Married (%)	Single (%)	Total (%)	Married (%)	Single (%)	Total (%)
(20-30)	13 (26%)	6 (12%)	19 (38%)	16 (32%)	4 (8%)	20 (40%)
(30-40)	22 (44%)	3 (6%)	25 (50%)	20 (40%)	8 (16%)	28 (56%)
(40-50)	6 (12%)	0 (0%)	6 (12%)	2 (4%)	0 (0%)	2 (4%)
Total	41 (82%)	9 (18%)	50 (100%)	38 (76%)	12 (24%)	50 (100%)

Table 1. Distribution of melasma percentage in females according to age and marital status.

3.2. Clinical response

Comparison between formulation treated group and placebo treated group indicated a significant differences for overall response to treatment. The improvement in active treatment group was 93% (40/43), while the corresponding value in placebo treated group was 4% (2/50), (P=0.001). Table 2. The effect of the formulated cream was demonstrated from the 1st week of treatment course (6.9%), with subsequent increase in improvement rate for week 2 (20.9%), week 3 (30.2%) and week 4 (34.8%)(P=0.007).

Variable		**Number improved [%]** Formulation [43 Patient]		Placebo [50 subject]		**P value**
		Weekly improved	Cumulative improvement	Weekly improved	**Cumulative improvement**	
Treatment period	Week 1	3 [6.9]	3 [6.9]	0 [0]	0 [0]	0.18
	Week 2	9 [20.9]	12 [27.9]	1 [2]	1 [2]	0.009
	Week 3	13 [30.2]	25 [58.13]	1 [2]	2 [4]	0.005
	Week 4	15 [34.8]	40 [93.00]	0 [0]	2 [4]	0.001
P value		0.007		0.58		
Total response [%]		40 [93]		2 [4]		0.001
No response [%]		3 [6.9]		48 [96]		

Table 2. Clinical results of studied and control females with melasma after treatment with the product.

Comparison between the active treated cream and placebo on week interval indicated anon significant improvement for the first week of the treatment course (P=0.18). However, there was a significant difference in the improvement rate between the two treatment groups for week 2 (P=0.009), week 3 (P=0.005) and week 4 (P=0.001), Table 2.

4. Discussion

This clinical trial indicated that 2.5% G. glabra cream was effective as treatment for melasma in a 28 days course with minimal side effects. However, this finding needs to be strengthening in a large scale clinical trial. Licorice is an extract with an important depigmenting property, obtained from *Glycyrrhiza glabra.* Known as "alcacus", it contains many compounds, of which saponins and flavonoids have the greatest antiphlogistic action [20]. In mouse cell culture, it was observed that Licorice has glabridine, the main component of the hydrophobic fraction of the extract, with the ability to inhibit tyrosinase without affecting DNA synthesis. The *in vivo* results were compatible with those *in vitro,* and immunohistochemical analysis showed a reduction of DOPA-positive melanocytes [21]. Moreover, Licorice has anti-inflammatory action by inhibiting some enzymes of the arachidonic acid cascade, especially cyclooxigenase, released after exposure to UV rays [22]. Due to these properties, glabridine is an important depigmenting component of the extract.

Nonetheless, Licorice has other components with depigmenting effects, such as liquiritin, which disperses melanin. In addition, Licorice has other active ingredient which exert antioxidant activity and thus Licorice cosmetic properties are attributed to its wide spectrum of antioxidant activity [23].Ultraviolet radiation in the skin leads to the formation of peroxides that induce the development of free radicals [24]. Certain licorice constituents possess significant antioxidant properties. Glycyrrhizin and glabridin inhibit the generation of reactive oxygen species (ROS) by neutrophils at the site of inflammation [6].

Traditionally, the use of depigmenting topical substances is without a doubt the best therapeutic option for the clinical treatment of melasma. Hydroquinone, although having some disadvantages, is the most used therapeutic alternative. [25,26] Nonetheless, many other substances, mostly of plant origin, have become more popular in dermatologic treatment [27]. In this study, the use of 2.5% *G. glabra* extract cream shows a reduction in melasma depending on digital evaluation and size of the lesion.

This study strengthens the clinical benefits of the *G. glabra* extract substances in the literature due to their melanin-dependent action (inhibiting tyrosinase, depleting or preventing the migration of melanosomes) and/or free radical-dependent action (melanogenic inhibition by preventing radical action on the melanocytes). The active group showed a reduction in the absolute number of lesions, according to the results obtained by digital photographic imaging, with significant statistical differences between the active and placebo group.

The adverse effects observed in both groups (Active and placebo) were well tolerated, spontaneously regressing with the use of the products. We observed, however, that these effects were less noticed in women using our formulation as only one lady developed allergic contact dermatitis. However, the side effect in the present study was less than that reported in subjects using hydroquinone (2%) [28]. Such data suggest the higher safety of *G. glabra* extract at 2.5% concentration product used by our patients as compared with hydroquinone, whose degree of tolerance has already been questioned in the literature [26,29].

The superiority of this greater depigmenting tendency could be better assessed in a prospective clinical study with a higher number of volunteers. Thus this study indicates that, depending on the concentrations used, plant extracts can be as efficient as hydroquinone in the treatment of melasma, without the side effect of hydroquinone. This confirms the viability of future competitive clinical studies to accurately elucidate a possible clinical superiority and ratify a tendency of higher tolerability of this new depigmenting alternative. In addition, combination of G. glabra extract with sun screen in a single formulated is recommended.

Author details

Amina Hamed Alobaidi[1*], Eqbal Salih Hamad[1,2], Abdulghani Mohamed Alsamarai[1] and Kudair Abass Kudair[1]

*Address all correspondence to: aminahamed2006@gmail.com

1 Departments of Biochemistry and Medicine, Tikrit University College of Medicine, Tikrit Teaching Hospital, Tikrit, Iraq

2 State Company for Drugs Industries, Samara, Salahuldean, Iraq

References

[1] Alsamarai AGM. Prevalence of skin diseases in Iraq. Int J Dermatol 2009; 48: 734-739.

[2] Ortonne JP, Arellano I, Berneburg M, Cestari T, Chan H, Grimes P, et al. A global survey of the role of ultraviolet radiation and hormonal influences in the development of melasma. J Eur Acad Dermatol Venereol. 2009;23:1254–1262.

[3] Olumide, Y. M. "Use of skin lightening creams".2010; BMJ 341 (nov23 2): c6102–c6102.

[4] Shabbir M, Khan MR, Saeed N. Assessment of phytochemicals, antioxidant, anti-lipid peroxidation and anti-hemolytic activity of extract and various fractions of Maytenus royleanus leaves. BMC Complement Altern Med. 2013 Jun 22;13:143. doi: 10.1186/1472-6882-13-143.

[5] Hikino H., Recent Research on Oriental Medicinal Plants, in Wagner H., Hikino H.,and Farnsworth NR. (eds.), Economic and medicinal Plant Research; London: Academic Press. 1, (53) 2003.

[6] Haraguchi H, Yoshida N, Ishikawa H, et al. Protection of mitochondrial functions against oxidative stresses by isoflavans from Glycyrrhiza glabra. J Pharm Pharmacol 2000;52:219-223.

[7] Chipault, J. R.; Mizuno, G. R.; Hawkins, J. M.; Lundberg, W.O. The antioxidant properties of natural spices. Food Res.2001, 17, 46-55.

[8] Olukoga A, Donaldson D. Historical perspectives on health. The history of liquorice: the plant, its extract, cultivation, and commercialisation and etymology. J R Soc Health 2001;118:300-304.

[9] Utsunomiya T, Kobayashi M, Pollard RB, Suzuki F. Glycyrrhizin, an active component of licorice roots. Plant Physiol, 2004;121:821-8.

[10] Mabberley, D. J. a Portable Dictionary of Plants, their Classification and Uses. Mabberley's Plant-book: 3rd Edition. Cambridge University Press, (2008).

[11] Hearing, V. J. The regulation of melanin production. Hori, W. eds.Drug Discovery Approaches for Developing Cosmeceuticals, Advanced Skin Care and Cosmetic Products.1997,3.1.1-3.1.21 IBC Library Series Southborough, Massachusetts.

[12] Kligman AM, Willis I. A new formula for depigmenting human skin. Arch Dermatol. 2005;111:40–8.

[13] Holliday, R. The extreme arrogance of anti-aging medicine. Biogerontology. 2009;10 (2): 223–8.

[14] Draelos ZD. Cosmetic therapy. In: Wolverton SE, editor. Comprehensive Dermatologic Drug Therapy. 2nd ed. Philadelphia: Saunders; 2007. pp. 761–74.

[15] Mayo Clinic: Moisturizers: Options for softer skin Dec. 16, 2010.

[16] Jung, H. W.; Tschaplinski, T. J.; Wang, L.; Glazebrook, J.; Greenberg, J. T. Priming in Systemic Plant Immunity. Science 2009; 5923: 89–91.

[17] Benchikhi H, Razoli H, Lakhdar H. Sunscreens: use in pregnant women in Casablanca. Ann Dermatol Venereol. 2002;129:387-90.

[18] Kochevar, I. E. Molecular and cellular effects of UV radiation relevant to chronic photodamage. Gilchrest, B. A. eds. Photodamage, 2001 ;51-67 Blackwell Science Cambridge, Massachusetts.

[19] Alobaidi AH, Hamad ES, Kudair KA, Alsamarai AGM. Formulation of Hypopigmentation Cream and Evaluation of its Effect on Skin Pigment. Part I: Formulation of the Product. Our Dermatol Online 2014;5:9-13.

[20] Yokota T, Nishio H, Kubota Y, Mizoguchi M. The inhibitory effect of glabridin from licorice extracts on melanogenesis and inflammation. Pigment Cell Res 1998;11:355-61.

[21] Zhu W, Gao J. The use of botanical extracts as topical skin lightening agents for the improvement of skin pigmentation disorders. J Investig Dermatol Symp Proc 2008;13:20-4.

[22] Hruza LL, Pentland AP. Mechanisms of UV induced inflammation. J Investig Dermatol 1993;100:35S-41S.

[23] Asl MN, Hosseinzadeh H. Review of pharmacological effects of Glycyrriza sp.and its bioactive compound. Phytother Res 2008;22:709-724.

[24] Heng CYM. Curcumin targeted signaling pathways: biasis for anti-photoaging and anti-carcinogenic therapy. Int J Dermatol 2010;49:608-622.

[25] Guevara IL, Pandya AG. Melasma treated with hydroquinone, tretinoin, and a fluorinated steroid. Int J Dermatol 2001;40:212-5.

[26] Draelos ZD. Cosmetic therapy. In: Wolverton SE, editor. Comprehensive Dermatologic Drug Therapy. 2nd ed. Philadelphia: Saunders; 2007. pp. 761–74.

[27] Lim JT. Treatment of melasma using kojic acid in a gel containing hydroquinone and glycolic acid. Dermatol Surg 1999;25:282-4.

[28] Zawar VP, Mhaskar ST. Exogenous ochronosis following hydroquinone for melasma. J Cosmet Dermatol. 2004;3:234–6.

[29] Mahé A, Ly F, Perret JL. Systemic complications of the cosmetic use of skin-bleaching products. Int J Dermatol 2005;44(Suppl 1):37-8.

Chapter 3

Evaluation of the Therapeutic Effect of Combined Conventional Asthma Drugs with Tianeptine in Treatment of Asthma — Double-Blind Controlled Trial Pilot Study

Abdulghani Mohamad Alsamarai,
Mohammad Ghiyath Alhelwani and
Amina Hamed Ahmed Alobaidi

Additional information is available at the end of the chapter

http://dx.doi.org/10.5772/58917

1. Introduction

Asthma is a chronic inflammatory and immunologic common which associated with reversable obstruction of airflow. Arab countries are with 20% prevalence rate and ambient air pollution may contribute to rise in this rate with time. Environmental factors are known to play an important role in the elicitation of asthma in genetically predisposed individuals. Although there has also been an increase in the awareness among doctors to diagnose asthma, a combination of various other factors may also be involved in the increased prevalence of asthma. Further investigations are recommended to identify the etiologic factors contributing to the rising prevalence of this disorder in Arab countries [1].

Asthma is common with an increasing prevalence and mortality especially in low-income and minority populations. The National Heart, Lung, and Blood Institute (NHLBI) defined asthma as *"recurrent episodes of respiratory symptoms; variable airflow obstruction that is often reversible, either spontaneously or with treatment; presence of airway hyper reactivity; and, importantly, chronic airway inflammation in which many cells and cellular elements play a role, in particular, mast cells, eosinophils, T- lymphocytes, macrophages, neutrophils, and epithelial cells"*[2]

Asthma is an important worldwide health priority because of its high and increasing prevalence, high morbidity and mortality, and direct and indirect costs. Asthma is with a prevalence of 12% of the population [3] with significant impact on quality of life and cost. [4]. The most important thing that relialized is asthma has been associated with significant comorbidities, especially depression [5-10]. Although stress triggered asthma symptoms, does not all of a sudden cause a person to develop the disease of asthma. [11,12]. The course of asthma appears to be influenced by mood and emotions and there is a high prevalence of depression or depressive symptoms in both children and adults with asthma.[11,12]

Recent studies indicated a positive association between stress and asthma exacerbation [13].

The chronicity of asthma course and episodic recurrences may lead to development of depression in asthmatic patients, specially in subjects with severe uncontrolled asthma [14]. Depression is associated with increased use of asthma-related urgent care services, emergency rooms, hospitals, and unscheduled appointments for asthma. as well as a variety of unfavorable asthma outcomes. Despite data on the frequency of depression in asthma and its adverse consequences, it is generally not recognized or treated.

Combination of conventional treatment drugs with antidepressants may amliorate asthma course and attack severity [15]. Both asthma and depression shared some biological linkage and antidepressant may be of therapeutic benefit through induction of bronchodilatation and reduction in cytokines production in asthmatic patients [16,17,18]. Immune and inflammatory responses in asthmatic patients may be modulated by antidepressants [18,19]. The ideal antidepressant to be used for treatment of asthma in combination with conventional drugs should have bronchodilator and anti-inflammatory activity and non-sedating such as tianeptine [20].

The present study was conducted to determine the therapeutic efficacy of Tianeptine in patients with asthma. Informed cosent taken from each subject included in the study and the study protocol was approved by the ethical committee.

Objectives: To determine the therapeutic efficacy of Tianeptine in patients with asthma.

2. Patients and methods

2.1. Study population

The study was performed on asthmatic patients. The subjects included in the study were recruited from the Habib Hospital outpatients Clinic in the Kingdom of Saudi Arabia. [Table 1]. The sample size in the study was 82 adult patients suffering from asthma for at least one year duration, and their age range was from 18 to 70 years, with a mean age of 35.8 years. The diagnosis and classification of asthma was performed by specialist physician and was established according to the National Heart Blood and Lung Institute / World Health Organization (NHLBI/WHO) workshop on the Global Strategy for Asthma [21]. The diseases severity classification was performed according to GIN criteria [22]. Patients were excluded if they were smokers, if they had malignancy, heart failure, history of venous embolisms, coronary heart disease and liver or kidney diseases..Current substance or alcohol Abuse/dependence, MDD with psychotic features (delusions, hallucinations, disorganized thought processes) or schizophrenia or schizoaffective disorder or if they had mental retardation or other severe cognitive impairment or if they were on current antipsychotic or antidepressant therapy or psychotherapy. Initiation of other psychotropic medications or psychotherapy within past 2 weeks (e.g., anxiolytics, hypnotics) and if they were pregnant or nursing women.

Group	Used drugs	Total numbers of patient in the group	Number of patients completed the trial	Average of patients age/yr Mean [SD]	Number of male patients	Number of female patients
1	Conventional	22	18	35.88 [14.02]	9	9
2	Conventional+ Tianeptine	21	15	36.4 [13.33]	8	7
3	Singulair+ Tianeptine	19	15	35.53 [12.72]	8	7
4	Conventiona+ fexofenadine+ Tianeptine	20	17	35.7 [10.85]	8	9
P value		NS	NS	NS	NS	NS

Table 1. Study population

Inclusion criteria includes: Out patients; Bronchial asthma has been known at least for 1 year ; Absene of long-term remissions of asthma (lasting more than 3 months) ; Poorly controlled asthma, due to various reasons ; No changes in asthma medications. ; and Both male and female

2.2. Study design

This study is randomized controlled trial to evaluate the therapeutic activity of tianeptine for treatment of asthma. The patients were distributed randomly to the groups. Patients who were eligible for entry in the study were included and follow-up for 8 weeks. Each patient had three visits, the first when introduce him\her in the study then the second after a month and the third was after two months

2.3. Measurement of stress

Perceived Stress Scale (PSS)[23] was used to measure the perception of stress in our study population. The Perceived Stress Scale is the only empirically established index of general stress appraisal. "The PSS measures the degree to which situations in one's life is appraised as stressful [24]. The PSS is not a diagnostic instrument, so there are no cut-offs. There are only comparisons between people in a given sample relationship between PSS scores and health behaviors and relationship among performance appraisal discomfort and belief, core self-evaluation and perceived stress.

There are three versions of the PSS: One with 4, one with 10, and one with 14 items. The 14-item version, which is the version that was adapted culturally to our study, as it had been used in previous studies and, at that time. Thus, the version we used has 14 items and is rated on a 5-point Liker type scale, ranging from 0 (*never*) to 4 (*very frequently*). Scores of items 4, 5, 6, 7, 9, 10, and 13 are reversed. Higher scores correspond to higher perceived stress. Internal consistency and factor structure data are mentioned in the introduction.[25]

2.4. Treatment schedule

The patients were distributed randomly into four groups each one include 25 patients. Selection of patients and distribution of them in the groups will be equally matched in gender, severity and presence of attack.

- **The first group** given conventional asthma treatment [SYMBICORT (budesonide and formoterol inhalation) or SEROTID (Salmeterol, fluticasone propionate).with or without salbutamol].
- **The second group** given conventional asthma treatment plus tianeptine12.5mg three times daily
- **The third group** given Singulair 10mg once daily (montelukast) plus tianeptine
- **The fourth group** is given conventional treatment with fexofenadine180 mg once daily plus tianeptine

2.5. Research methodolog

a. After making sure of the status of each individual from the patients have asthma and they are eligible for this study design and did not have any of the exceptions for the study will be admitted to one of the study groups. Informed written consent taken from all patients included in the study.

b. Baseline assessment conducted for each patient at the time of enrollment in the study,also recording the number of attacks suffered by the patient during the week and the number of times where he \she wake up because of shortness of breath and the number of times sprays ventolen during the week and the number of absences from school or work during the month due to asthma and assessing the severity of cough and the severity of breathing difficulty suffered by the patient that were divided to three degrees,simple, moderate and severe. Also study and record presence of wheezing or not. As spirometry remains an essential diagnostic tool in assessment of asthmatic patient But we will limit ourselves to study Peak Expiratory Flow Rate (PEFR) because it is a simple method of measuring airway obstruction the device is available, accessible, and easy to use by the patient and it will detect moderate or severe disease. The simplicity of the method is its main advantage. It is measured using a standard Wright Peak Flow Meter or mini Wright Meter. The needle must always be reset to zero before PEF is measured. The measurement of peak expiratory flow rate (PEFR) three to four times allows the diagnosis and assessment of the severity of asthma. [26]. It will be studied for all patients, and the stress and anxiety status of patients will determined for all patients included in the study by using Perceived Stress Scale. Arabic version of the questions set prepared and used through the study.

c. Patients evaluation performed at interval of the study and at least to attend the chest clinic 3 times during the study period.

Visit 1: Screening visit:

The following actions were taken

- take the written consent of the patient on the study after explaining all matters relating thereto
- General medical history & physical examination.
- Study of stress and anxiety status by Complete Perceived Stress Scale
- Measure peak expiratory flow
- Complete asthma control questionnaire.

Visit 2: 4weeks after visit 1

The following actions were taken

- Baseline clinical measurements
- Complete asthma control questionnaire
- Measure peak expiratory flow

Visit 3: 4weeks after visit 2

Repeat all the actions taken in the visit 2

At each study visit the peak expiratory flow (PEF) will be performed, the best of three measurements will be recorded [27].

2.6. Asthma control questionnaire

International guidelines for the treatment of asthma have identified that the primary clinical goal of asthma management is to optimise asthma control (minimisation of symptoms, activity limitation, and bronchoconstriction and rescue β_2 -agonist use) and thus reduce the risk of life-threatening exacerbations and long-term morbidity. The Asthma Control Questionnaire (ACQ) was developed to meet these criteria. It measures both the adequacy of asthma control and change in asthma control, which occurs either spontaneously or as a result of treatment [28]. We have developed a schedule for each patient where the following questions is registered for all visits to facilitate consideration of the patient's condition fully [29].

1. In the past 4 weeks, how much of the time did your asthma keep you from getting as much done at work, school or at home?
2. During the past 4 weeks, how often have you had attacks of shortness of breath?
3. During the past 4 weeks, how often did your asthma symptoms (wheezing, coughing, and shortness of breath, chest tightness or pain) wake you up at night or earlier than usual in the morning?
4. During the past 4 weeks, how often have you used your rescue inhaler or nebulizer medication (such as salbutamol)?
5. Assessment of severity of cough, SOB.
6. Is there wheezing or no?
7. How would you rate your asthma control during the past 4 weeks?
8. Recording peak expiratory flow

2.7. Statistical analysis

SPSS package (version 17) was used for statistical analysis.

3. Results

Out of the total (82) patients with asthma included in the study, 79% (65 patients) of them continued until the end of the study and are eligiable for analysis. The subjects suitable for analysis are consisted of 33 men (52%) and 32 women (48%). The mean age was 35.8 years (Table 1).

3.1. Role of conventional asthma treatment in the first group

In this study 22 patients has been selected for the first group, 18 patients (81.8%) of them continued until the end of the study. Of the total, 9 patients were male and 9 were female and they were given conventional asthma treatment only [SYMBICORT (budesonide and formoterol inhalation) or SEROTID (Salmeterol, fluticasone propionate) with or without salbutamol]. Their results are shown in Table 3. The average age of patients was 35.8 year, average severity of symptoms was 2.78, medication score was 3.94 and PSS value was 22.94. There was significant clinical impact of ventolin, Symbicort and Seretide conventional in treatment of asthma. Then average of improvement after a month was 1.94 and increased to 2.11 after 2 months period (P= 0.001) from the base line and PEFR increased from 72.6% at the time of enrollement in the study to 83.6% at the end of the study (P=0.0001).

Variable		Mean	Std. Deviation	Std. Error Mean	95% Confidence interval
Age		35.89	14.02	3.31	28.92 – 42.86
Severity of asthma		2.78	1.26	0.30	2.15 – 3.41
Medication score		3.94	1.80	0.42	3.04 – 4.83
PSS Score		22.94	7.90	1.86	19.01 – 26.87
Rate of improvement	1 month	1.93	0.24	0.06	1.74-2.13
	2 month	2.11	0.47	0.11	1.83 – 2.39
	P value	0.001			
PEFR	Study onset	72.67	10.69	2.52	67.35 – 77.99
	End of the study	83.61	8.63	2.16	79.3 – 87.9
	P value	0.0001			

Table 2. Combined rates of all data for patients of Conventional treatment (group 1)

3.2. Role of conventional asthma treatment plus Tianeptine in the second group

These patients were given the same of traditional medicines which given to the first group, but was added Tianeptine to each patients in this group. The average patients age was 36.4 year, average severity of symptoms was 3.06, medication score was 3.9 and PSS value was 22.33. The treatment lead to improvement of 1.93 after a month and this increased to 2.4 after 2 months with significant difference (P= 0.001) from the baseline. In addition, PEFR increased from 77.4% at study enrollement to 89.13% at the end of the study (P= 0.0001).

Variable		Mean	Std. Deviation	Std. Error Mean	95% onfidence interval
Age		36.40	13.33	3.44	29.03 – 43.76
Severity of asthma		3.07	.96	.25	2.54 – 3.60
Medication score		4.73	1.44	.37	3.93 – 5.53
PSS score		22.33	7.79	2.01	18.03 – 26.63
Rate of improvement	1 month	1.93	.258	.067	1.74-2.13
	2 month	2.40	.63	.16	2.09-2.70
	P value	0.001			
PEFR	Study onset	77.40	7.88	2.03	73.05 – 81.75
	End of study	89.13	4.88	1.26	86.43 – 91.83
	P value	0.0001			

Table 3. Combined rates of all data for patients of Conventional treatment with Tianeptine [group 2]

3.3. Role of Tianeptine ± Singulair in asthmath in the third group

These patients were given Tianeptine12.5+Singulair10mg without addition or modification of traditional medicines. The average of patient's age was 35.53, average severity of symptoms was 2.46, medication score was 6, and average of PSS of this group was 23.06. The improvement after a month was 1.00 and increased to 2.13 after 2 months (P=0.001) from the baseline. Furthermore, average of Rate of peak expiratory flow at onset of study was 80.4% and increased to 88.4% at the end of the study (P=0.001).

Variable		Mean	SD	St. Error of mean	95% confidence interval
Age		35.53	12.72	3.28	28.50 – 42.56
Severity of asthma		2.47	0.92	0.24	1.96 – 2.98
Medication score		6.00	0.00	0.00	6.00 – 6.00
PSS score		23.07	5.88	1.52	19.82 – 26.32
Rate of improvement	1 month	1.00	0.38	0.10	0.81-1.19
	2 month	2.13	0.74	0.19	1.83-2.44
	P value	0.001			
PEFR	Study onset	80.40	5.55	1.43	77.33 – 83.47
	End of study	88.40	7.34	1.89	83.34 – 92.46
	P value	0.001			

Table 4. Combined rates of all data for patients of Singulair with Tianeptine [group3]:

3.4. Role of conventional medicines ± fexofenadine ± tianeptine in asthma in the fourth group

In this group, 17 patients continued until the end of the study, including 8 patients were male and 9 were female. The patients were given the same of traditional medicines given to the first group, but was added Tianeptine (12.5 mg) three time daily and fexofenadine (180 mg) once daily to each patients in this group. Average of patient's age of fourth group was 35.7, average of severity of symptoms was 3.17, medication score was 7, and average of PSS of this group was 26.67. The average of improvement after a month was 2.41and this increased to 2.58 after 2 month of treatment (P=0.0001). In addition, PEFR was increased to 88.41% at the end of the study (P=0.0001)

Variable		Mean	Std. Deviation	Std. Error Mean	95% Confidence interval
Age		35.71	10.85	2.63	30.13 – 41.29
Severity of asthma		3.18	1.42	.35	2.45 – 3.91
Medication score		7.00	.00	.00	7.00 – 7.00
PSS score		26.65	4.65	1.13	24.26 – 29.04
Rate of improvement	1 month	2.41	.51	.12	2.23 - 2.59
	2 month	2.59	.51	.12	2.30-2.89
	P value	0.001			
PEFR	Study onset	73.29	7.99	1.94	69.18 – 77.40
	End of study	88.41	7.50	1.82	84.55 – 92.27
	P value	0.0001			

Table 5. Combinee rates of all data for patients of Conventional treatment with Fexofenadine + Tianeptine [group 4]:

3.5. Comparison between the rates of the key points for all groups

The averages of PSS for all groups were roughly convergent (P>0.05). All patients in the four groups have made improvement with lightly varying degrees in the first month, with the exception of the third group. However, the percentage of improvement in patients of this group in the first month was relatively low, but after two months the improvement became well. Furthermore, the average improvement after a month of treatment course was with highly significant differences between the groups (P=0.000). However, the average improvement after 2 month was with non significant differences between the groups (P=0.06). The same pattern of differences was achieved for PEFR, however, the changes in PEFR were significantly different between the groups. Although the severity of asthma was more in group 4, the increase change was more prominent in this group as compared to other 3 groups.Table 6.

Variable	Improvement		PEFR Percent		
	After 1 month	After 2 month	PEFR 1	PEFR 2	Change
Group 1	1.94	2.11	72.66	83.61	10.95
Group 2	1.93	2.40	77.40	89.13	11.73
Group 3	1.00	2.13	80.40	88.40	08.00
Group 4	2.41	2.58	73.20	88.41	15.21
P value ANOVA	0.000	0.067	0.034	>0.05	<0.05

Improvment1: Mean rate of overall improvement in the group after the first month

Improvment2: Mean rate of overall improvement in the group after the second month

PEFR1: Mean rate of peak expiratory flow of the group at the beginning of the study

PEFR2: Mean rate of peak expiratory flow of the group at the end of the study

Change: Mean the difference between the rate of peak expiratory flow between the beginning and end of the study

Table 6. Improvement comparison between the treatment groups

The proportion of decreasing of the mean percentage change of daily "as-needed" inhaled β-agonist using for patients of each group were 25.5%, 31.1%, 26.6% and 35.8% for groups1,2,3,and 4 respectively. The present study demonstrated non significant differences in proportion of decreasing between the 4 groups. However, all groups demonstrated significant differences in proportion of decreasing inhaled β-agonist use at the end of the study as compared to enrollement time. Table 7.

Variable	Number	Difference number of salbutamol using between onset and end study				P value
		Mean	SD	95% Confidence interval	Rate of decrease	
Group 1	18	2.56	2.57	1.27 - 3.83	25.5%	0.001
Group 2	15	3.13	1.58	2.86 - 4.61	31.1%	0.000
Group 3	15	2.67	1.05	2.09 - 3.25	26.6%	0.000
Group 4	17	3.59	1.94	2.59 - 4.58	35.8%	0.000
P value ANOVA		>0.05			>0.05	

Table 7. Proportion of decreasing of the mean percentage change of daily "as-needed" inhaled β-agonist using for patients of for treatment groups

In conclusion, the 4 treatment course were effective therapeutic approaches for asthma treatment, however, the combination of SYMBICORT (budesonide and formoterol inhalation) or SEROTID (Salmeterol, fluticasone propionate) plus Tianeptine (12.5 mg) three time daily and fexofenadine (180 mg) once daily was superior in treating severe asthma.

4. Discussion

Individuals with asthma have twice the risk of developing mood and anxiety disorders as individuals without asthma and these psychological factors are associated with worse outcomes and greater need for medical intervention. Similarly, asthma symptom onset and exacerbation often occur during times of increased psychological stress. Remission from depression, on the other hand, is associated with improvement in asthma symptoms and decreased usage of asthma medication. Yet research aimed at understanding the biological underpinnings of asthma has focused almost exclusively on the periphery. An extensive literature documents the relationship between emotion and asthma, but little work has explored the function of affective neural circuitry in asthma symptom expression.[30]

The present study indicated that in patients receiving Tianeptine plus conventional asthma treatment (group 2) demonstrate a hsigigher decrease in the mean percentage change in daily "as-needed" inhaled β-agonist use (31.1%) as compared to patients group receiving conventional asthma treatment (group 1) only (25.5%). Also, there was a higher decrease in the mean percentage change in daily "as-needed" inhaled β-agonist use (35.8%) in the fourth group which given conventional treatment with fexofenadine plus tianeptine as compared to the other 3 groups of treatment. However, using ANOVA analysis, the differences in percentage change in daily "as –needed" between the four groups were not statistically significant. Furthermore, the percentage of change was highly significant for the four groups of treatment.

PEFR was improved significantly in the four groups, however, there was a significant differences in changes between the four ngroups of treatment. Furthermore, the PEFR change was more in group four (conventional + tianeptine + fexofenadine) and lowest in group 3 (singulair plus Tianeptine). The rate of improvement was highest in group 4 and lowest in group 3 after one month of treatment course and the there was a highly significant differences between the 4 groups in their rate of improvement. However, after 2 months of treatment there was no significant differences between the groups in their rate of improvement. This could be explasined on the basis that fexofenadine may exert antiinflammatory action that may influence the clinical improvement [31-38]

In this study the impact of Tianeptine was clear through the big improvement in patients who receice this medicine, as demonstrated in reduction of daily use and percent reduction of salbutamol, percent changes in PEFR and rate of improvement in group 2,3 and 4. However, the above parameters changes were lower in group of patients (group 3) receiving singulair with Tianeptine. This could be due to that singulair acts as antiinflammatory, it does prevent bronchoconstriction, but not relieve the present bronchoconstriction. In addition, it takes 3 -4 to reach high peak blood mean (Tmax)[39].

The therapeutic effect of Tianeptine in treatment of asthma may be contributed to its ability to suppress proinflammatory cytokines, interference with cholinergic and serotoninergic pathways, modulation of immune response and/or serotonin uptake by platelets and serotonergic axons at the central nervous system [40,41]. Serotonin induces bronchoconstriction via peripheral and central pathways resulting in increasing colinergic activity and histamine release[42]. These changes may explain why tianeptine has proven to be a powerful therapeutic tool in controlling asthma as this study indicated of better improvement in groups (groups 2,3,and 4) receiving tinaneptine. During asthma attack, catacholamines and free serotonin (f-5-HT), only f-5-HT levels correlated positively with pulmonary function clinical severity [43,44]. f-5-HT was taken up by pulmonary endocrine cells that were located at the parasympathetic terminals. Pulmonary endocrine cells located at the parasympathetic terminals taken up f-5-HT. Bronchial smooth muscle contracted due to effect of serotonin through potententiation of acetylcholine [39]. However, postsynaptic receptors (5-HT3 and 5-HT4) that located at the bronchial muscle mediated serotonin effects.

A reported studies [45,46] suggested that tinaneptine therapy reduce plasma f-5-HT, clinical rating and increase in pulmonary function. While, asthma attach triggered by drugs that increase f-5HT such as buspirone and serotonin-uptake inhibitors (like sertraline, paroxetine, etc).[47-50]. However, the side effects of buspirone and serotonin inhibitors may be controlled by atropine [51]. Dupon et al.[52] suggested that serotonin produced frequency- and concentration-dependent facilitation of cholinergic contractions of human airways, which was mimicked by both 5-HT_3 and 5-HT_4 agonists, and subsequently 5-HT facilitates cholinergic contractions in the human airways. In addition, Tianeptine greatlly annulated pulmonary vasoconstriction and bronchoconstriction that induced by drugs through their ability to increase f-5HT serum levels [53-59]. Neuroepithelial autocrine serotonergic cells located at the bronchopulmonary system release 5-HT under the effect of acetylcholine stimulation, while, serotonin triggers acetylcholine release from the parasympathetic terminals [60].

Mood disordera are more common in individuals with atopy [13]. Through our study, we can say Tianeptine definitely seems to improve the asthma as it reduced the severity of symptoms and improved the daily functioning of a asthmatic patient and reduced absences from school or work, with increase PEFR, whether that it was added to traditional medicines (budesonide and formoterol inhalation or Salmeterol, fluticasone propionate)or Singulair or fexofenadine. But Group who took the traditional medicines for asthma with the addition of tianeptine and fexofenadine was better and their symptoms responded to treatment better than others. This finding may be due to synergistic antiinflamatory effects that induced by combination of Tianeptine and fexofenadine.

Tianeptine led to a clinical improvement of asthmatic symptoms in the second group, patients who were given the tianeptine in addition to traditional medicine has with better improvement as compared to the first group who took traditional medicines only. This suggests the positive effect of this drug for patients with asthma, of course not as a single medicine, but certainly as adjuvant drug to the essential approved medicines. The mechanism by which this positive impact was induced may be due to its significant anxiolytic properties for patients with asthma who worry more than others or due to positive association between free serotonin in plasma and severity of asthma in symptomatic patients. As tianeptine was the only agent known to both reduce free serotonin in plasma and enhance uptake in platelets,[45,46]. Previous studies have shown that antidepressants may be of therapeutic value in asthma [61,62] as there is increasing evidence that a biological linkage may exist between asthma and depression [61,63,64]. A defect in the function of the autonomic nervous system such as alpha-adrenergic and cholinergic hyperresponsiveness and beta-adrenergic hyporesponsiveness even distal from the airways has been demonstrated in asthmatic patients, as well as in depression [61,64]. Antidepressants may have a therapeutic role in asthma by supressing proinflammatory cytokines and preventing their brain effects [61,65]. They also interfere with cholinergic and serotoninergic pathways, both centrally and peripherally. Most antidepressants also induce adaptive changes in central monoaminergic neurotransmission, which itself might modulate immune reactivity [61,65]. Tianeptine is an antidepressant drug that has been recently used with success in the treatment of asthma. Tianeptine treats depression through the enhancement of serotonin reuptake from the synaptic cleft by serotoninergic terminals. It works by a mechanism that is just the pollar opposite of selective serotonin reuptake inhibition. It has been reported that this substance provoked a dramatic disappearance of clinical symptoms and improved the pulmonary function in asthmatic patients [61,66].

Without the slightest doubt, the modern conventional medicine such as SYMBICORT (budesonide and formoterol inhalation) or SEROTID (Salmeterol, fluticasone propionate has provided great benefit for patients with asthma and It shall be the basis of good treatment for asthmatic patients in various degrees and severity. In the present study, these drugs had good results and improved symptoms of patient and their live quality. These treatment approach showed improvement in PEFR from 72.6% to 83.7%, with difference in the amount of 11% and significant decrease in the mean percentage change in daily "as-needed" inhaled β-agonist use of about 25%. Some randomised controlled trial comparing stable dose Seretide with Symbicort, given as an adjustable maintenance dose, in 706 adults with persistent asthma [67]. Over one year, those taking Serotide experienced the equivalent of 24 more symptom-free days compared to those taking symbicort. The overall incidence of asthma exacerbations (a severe attack) was 47% lower in the Seretide group. Overall, the majority of exacerbations did not result in hospitalisation. Morning peak expiratory flow was significantly higher with Seretide and those taking Seretide experienced a significantly higher proportion of days free of rescue medication use [67].

In the present study, the two drugs had similar results in controling asthma and these results were better in group 4 (given conventional treatment with fexofenadine plus tianeptine). As table 6 shows the extent of improvement after 2 months of treatment comparison between the four groups, the improvement of patients in fourth group was significant. This finding support existence of the synergistic role of fexofenadine with tianeptine and conventional asthma treatment, where the improvement in PEFR was greater in fourth group patients who took the both of drugs together with conventional course. In addition to traditional medicine fexofenadine has been shown to have an impact on inflammatory mediators, other than histamine, such as decreasing the production of LTC_4, LTD_4, LTE_4, PGE_2, and $PGF_{2\alpha}$; and diminishing eosinophil adherence, chemotaxis, and opsonization of particles.[68] These effects may provide benefit to some of the inflammatory responses of an acute allergic reaction and provide a basis for future development of H1 antagonists with stronger anti-inflammatory effects.[68]

Repeated dosing with fexofenadine (180mg) and montelukast (10 mg) as add-on therapy improved AMP PC20 and other surrogate inflammatory markers along with asthma diary outcomes in ICS-treated atopic asthmatic patients. [69]. However, in our study the patients of third group [given Singulair (montelukast) plus Tianeptine] were less responsive and less improved compared with other groups especially in the first month. This may be due to the combination of Singulair (montelukast) plus tianeptine only without the addition of drugs such as SYMBICORT or SEROTID. However, results of imrovement in group thee at the end of second month was better compared with the same group in the first month. This confirms preventive influence of Singulair, Montelukast in a long term-controller medication which should not be substituted for short acting β-agonists. Furthermore, this finding suggest not to use Singulair alone and to be used in combination with other prophylactic agent.

Montelukast is a preventive agent, which should be used in addition to other drugs for the management of asthma. [39] Therefore, as it is well known and previously confirmed, montelukast is effective as prophylactic drug and control of chronic asthmatic course for subjects aged ≥ 15 years, however, of no value as rescue treatment approach in acute attacks.[39]

The clinical benefit from adding Tianeptine to asthma therapy course may actually result in new indications for antidepressants. They could also help in understanding some common pathophysiological mechanisms existing between asthma and depression.[19]

The treatment for asthma and depression involves a coordinated approach that monitors both the symptoms of asthma and depression including using an asthma action plan. It is important to find the treatment that works best for each person. The most effective treatments are those that combine psychological and medical care, medical monitoring, individualised asthma education and adequate community support. It should be noted that while antidepressants seem to have no specific effect on asthma symptoms or medication, the National Asthma Council recommends that people should not take sedatives when having an acute attack of asthma as it may have an effect on breathing [70]

The natural course of asthma include a scenario of triggering phase followed by generation of symptom and inflammation phase to form a vicious cycle of subsequent phases [71]. Constitutional predisposition to the development of neurogenic generator component is necessary for asthma development. Although stress does not cause asthma, stress and asthma are definitely linked. Asthma causes stress, and stress makes it more difficult to control asthma. Even daily stress can make asthma symptoms worsen. The learning to change stress response to decrease asthma symptoms is important. Equally important is prioritizing patient daily schedule so he allow enough time to accomplish what the patient needs to do without feeling pressured or overwhelmed [71]

The study limitation is the small numbers of patients in each group. However, the power analysis calculated to determine the effect of sample size in each group. The power of analysis was 0.89 for reduction in PEFR for all groups, while that of rate improvement were 0.54 for group 2, 0.10 for group 3 and 0.72 for group 4. These findings indicated that sample size with influence on the finding of group 3 only. However, the power of analysis for the differences between the groups indicated a values of >0.97 for the 4 groups indicating non influence of sample sizes on the results.

In conclusion, the present study indicated the therapeutic activity of Tianeptine as add on drug in asthma control and treatment. The most effective combination course is that of fexofenadine, Tianeptine and conventional beta agonist such as symbicort or serotid. Until today, management of bronchial asthma was held in two main directions:Modification of factors inducing allergic reaction and interference on the certain stages of allergic reaction; and Interference with peripheral bronchial receptors. Both these directions do finally affect the trigger factors. Based on the present study findings, We suggest a 3rd direction in the management of bronchial asthma: application of antidepresion agents for the control of activity of generator neurogenic mechanisms of bronchial asthma. This new approach leads to the prevention of asthmatic attacks and opens up new perspectives for the management of this disease

Author details

Abdulghani Mohamad Alsamarai[2,3*], Mohammad Ghiyath Alhelwani[1] and Amina Hamed Ahmed Alobaidi[1]

*Address all correspondence to: galsamarrai@yahoo.com

1 Department of Medicine, Tikrit University College of Medicine, Tikrit, Iraq; College of Applied Medical Sciences, Netherland

2 Asthma and Allergy Centre, Tikrit Teaching Hospital, Tikrit, Iraq

3 Habib Hospital Outpatients Clinic, Saudi Arabia

Department of Biochemistry, Tikrit University College of Medicine, Tikrit, Iraq

References

[1] Al Frayh AR; Shakoor Z, Gad El Rab MO, Hasnain SM. Increased prevalence of asthma in Saudi Arabia. Ann Allergy Asthma Immunol. 2001 Mar;86(3):292-6.

[2] Global Initiative for Asthma. Global strategy for asthma management and prevention. NHLBI/WHO Workshop Report. NIH Publication 02-3659. Bethesda, MD: NHLBI, 2002.

[3] Ruffin R, Wilson D, Smith B, et al. Prevalence, morbidity and management of adult asthma in South Australia. *Immunol Cell Biol* 2001; 79: 191-194.

[4] Adams R, Wakefield M. Quality of life in asthma: a comparison of community and hospital asthma patients. *J Asthma* 2001; 38: 205-214.

[5] Serra-Batlles J, Plaza V, Morejun E, et al. Costs of asthma according to degree of severity. *Eur Respir J* 1998; 12: 1322-1326.

[6] Von Behren J, Kreutzer R, Hernandez A. Self-reported asthma prevalence in adults in California. *Asthma* 2002; 39: 429-440.

[7] Mancuso CA, Rincon M, McCulloch CE, Charlson ME. Selfefficacy, depressive symptoms,and patients' expectation predict outcomes in asthma. *Med Care* 2001; 39: 1326-1338.

[8] Rimington LD, Davies DH, Lowe D, Pearson MG. Relationship betweeen anxiety, depression, and morbidity in adult asthma patients. *Thorax* 2001; 56: 266-271.

[9] Manocchia M, Keller S, Ware JE. Sleep problems, healthrelated quality of life, work functioning and health care utilisation among the chronically ill. *Qual Life Res* 2001; 10: 331 345.

[10] Young SY, Gunzenhauser JD, Malone KE, McTiernan A.Body mass index and asthma in the military population of the northwestern United States. *Arch Intern Med* 2001; 161: 1605-1611.

[11] Van Lieshout RJ, Glenda MacQueen. Psychological Factors in Asthma. Allergy, Asthma, and Clinical Immunology, Vol 4, No 1 (Spring), 2008: pp 12–28

[12] Krommydas G, Gourgoulianis G, Raftopoulos V, Kotrotsiou E: Antidepressants And Asthma Treatment. The Internet Journal of Pulmonary Medicine. 2006 Volume 6 Number 1

[13] Alsamarai AGM. Influence of stress on exacerbation of asthma. Ann Iraqi Sci 2009;2:765-771.

[14] Tousman, Stuart. Asthma and Depression. Allergy and Asthma Advocate. Winter 2003. American Academy of Allergy Asthma & Immunology (AAAAI). 5 Nov. 2007. aaaai.org.

[15] Sugihara H, Ishihara K,Nogughi H:Clinical experience with amitriptyline (tryptanol) in the treatment of bronchial asthma Annals of Allergy 1965 ;23:422-429

[16] Krommydas G, Gourgoulianis KI, Angelopoulos N, Kotrotsiou E, Raftopoulos V, Molyvdas P-A. Depression and pulmonary function in outpatients with asthma. Resp Med 2004;98:220-24.

[17] Wright JR, Rodriguez M, Cohen S: Review of psychosocial stress and asthma: an intergrated biopsychosocial approach. Thorax 1998;53:1066 - 1074

[18] Krommydas G, Gourgoulianis KI, Karamitsos K, Krapis K, Molyvdas PA Therapeutic value of antidepressants in asthma. Med Hypotheses.2004 ;64:938-40

[19] Lechin F, van der Dijs B, Lechin AE.Treatment of bronchial asthma with Tianeptine. Methods Find Exp Clin Pharmacol.2004 ; 26 :1-5

[20] Zoladz PR, Muñoz C and Diamond DM. Beneficial Effects of Tianeptine on Hippocampus-Dependent Long-Term Memory and Stress-Induced Alterations of Brain Structure and Function *Pharmaceuticals* 2010; *3:* 3143-3166; doi:10.3390/ph3103143

[21] National Heart Lung and Blood Institute. Guidelines for the Diagnosis and Management of Asthma (EPR3). July 2007.

[22] Asthma GINA classification. 2008. http://www.slideshare.net/crisbertc/asthma-gina-classification

[23] Cohen, S. and Williamson, G. Perceived Stress in a Probability Sample of the United States. Spacapan, S. and Oskamp, S. (Eds.) *The Social Psychology of Health.* Newbury Park, CA: Sage, 1988.

[24] Cohen, S., Kamarck, T., and Mermelstein, R. A global measure of perceived stress. *Journal of Health and Social Behavior,1983; 24:* 386-396.

[25] Ramirez MTG, Hernadeze RL. Factor structure of Perceived Stress Scale (PSS) in a sample from mexico. The spenish Journal of Psychology 2007;10:199-206

[26] Cowie, RL, Revitt, SG, Underwood, MF, Field, SK. The effect of a peak flow-based action plan in the prevention of exacerbations of asthma. Chest 1997; 112:1534.

[27] Gildea TR, McCarthy K. Pulmonary function test. August, 2010. http://www.clevelandclinicmeded.com/medicalpubs/diseasemanagement/pulmonary/pulmonary-function-testing/

[28] Juniper's E. Measurme nt of Quality Health Life and Asthma Control. www.qol-tech.co.uk.

[29] American Lung Association. https://www.nationaljewish.org/NJH/media/pdf/pdf-Childhood_ACT.pdf]:

[30] Rosenkranz MA, Davidson RJ. Affective neural circuitry and mind–body influences in asthma. NeuroImage 2009;47:972–980

[31] Gelfand EW, Cui ZH, Takeda K, *et al*. Fexofenadine modulates T-cell function, preventing allergen-induced airway inflammation and hyperresponsiveness. J Allergy Clin Immunol 2002;110:85-95

[32] de Paulis A, Dente V, Onorati AM, *et al*. Fexofenadine inhibits the release of mediators and IL-4 from human FC, RI+ cells. Allergy 1999;54(Suppl 52):278

[33] Paolieri F, Battifora M, Riccio AM, *et al*. Terfenadine and fexofenadine reduce *in vitro* ICAM-1 expression on human continuous cell lines. Ann Allergy Asthma Immunol 1998;81:601-7

[34] Amon U, Amon S, Gibbs BF. *in vitro* studies with fexofenadine, a new nonsedating histamine H_1 receptor antagonist, on isolated human basophils [Abstr]. Inflamm Res 2000;49 (Suppl 1):S13-14

[35] Schroeder JT, Schleimer RP, Lichtenstein LM, *et al*. Inhibition of cytokine generation and mediator release by human basophils treated with desloratadine. Clin Exp Allergy 2001;31:1369-77

[36] Lippert U, Kruger-Krasagakes S, Moller A, *et al*. Pharmacological modulation of IL-6 and IL-8 secretion by the H_1-antagonist descarboethoxy-loratadine and dexamethasone by human mast and basophilic cell lines. Exp Dermatol 1995;4:272-6

[37] Genovese A, Patella V, De Crescenzo G, *et al*. Loratadine and desethoxylcarbonyl-loratadine inhibit the immunological release of mediators from human $Fc\varepsilon RI^+$ cells. Clin Exp Allergy 1997;27:559-67

[38] Geha RS, Meltzer EO. Desloratadine: a new, nonsedating, oral antihistamine. J Allergy Clin Immunol 2001;107:751-62

[39] Singulair clinical pharmacology http://www.healthscout.com/rxdetail/68/68/5/main.html, retrived 16/02/2012

[40] Krommydas G, Gourgoulianis KI, Karamitsos K, Krapis K, Molyvdas PA Therapeutic value of antidepressants in asthma. Med Hypotheses.2004 ;64:938-40]

[41] Lechin F, van der Dijs B, Lechin AE. Treatment of bronchial asthma with tianeptine. Methods Find Exp Clin Pharmacol. 2004 Nov;26(9):697-701].

[42] Lechin F, van der Dijs B, Lechin AE.Treatment of bronchial asthma with Tianeptine. Methods Find Exp Clin Pharmacol.2004 ; 26 :1-5

[43] Lechin, AE, Varon, J, van der Dijs, B, et al Plasma catecholamines and indoleamines during attacks and remission on severe bronchial asthma: possible role of stress [abstract].Am J Respir Crit Care Med 1994;149:A778

[44] Lechin, F, van der Dijs, B, Orozco, B, et al Increased levels of free-serotonin in plasma of symptomatic asthmatic patients. Ann Allergy Asthma Immunol 1996;77:245-253

[45] Lechin, F, van der Dijs, B, Orozco, B, et al Neuropharmacological treatment of bronchial asthma with an antidepressant drug: tianeptine; a double-blind crossover placebo-controlled study. Clin Pharmacol Ther 1998;64:223-232

[46] Lechin, F, van der Dijs, B, Lechin, A, et al The serotonin uptake-enhancing drug tianeptine suppresses asthmatic symptoms in children: a double-blind crossover placebo-controlled study. J Clin Pharmacol 1998;38:918-925.

[47] Lechin F, vander Dijs B, Lechin AB. Tianeptine : a new explorary for therapy for asthma. Chest 2004;125:348-349.

[48] Lechin, F, van der Dijs, B, Jara, H, et al. Effects of buspirone on plasma neurotransmitters in healthy subjects. J Neural Transm 1998;105:561-573

[49] Lechin, F, van der Dijs, B, Jackubowicz, D, et al. Role of stress in the exacerbation of chronic illness: effects of clonidine administration on blood pressure and plasma norepinephrine, cortisol, growth hormone and prolactin concentrations. Psychoneuroendocrinology 1987;12:117-129

[50] Lechin, F, van der Dijs, B, Orozco, B, et al Plasma neurotransmitters,blood pressure and heart rate during supine resting, orthostasis and moderate exercise in severely ill patients: a model of failing to cope with stress. Psychother Psychosom 1996;65:129-136

[51] Lechin, F, van der Dijs, B, Orozco, B, et al Plasma neurotransmitters, blood pressure and heart rate during supine-resting, orthostasis and moderate exercise stress test in healthy humans before and after parasympathetic blockade with atropine. Res Comm Biol Psychol Psychiatry 1996;21:55-72

[52] Dupont, LJ, Pype, JL, Dernedts, MG, et al. The effects of 5-HT on cholinergic contraction in human airways in vitro. Eur Respir J 1999;14:642-649

[53] Lechin, F, van der Dijs, B Serotonin and pulmonary vasoconstriction [letter]. J Appl Physiol 2002;92:1363-1364

[54] Lechin, F, van der Dijs, B, Lechin, AE. Pulmonary hypertension, left ventricular dysfunction and plasma serotonin [letter]. Br J Pharmacol 2002;137:937-938

[55] Lechin, F Asthma, asthma medication and autonomic nervous system dysfunction [letter]. Clin Physiol 2001;6:723

[56] Lechin, F, van der Dijs, B, Lechin, AE. Serotonin, pulmonary hypertension and bronchial asthma [letter]. Clin Sci 2002;103:345-346

[57] Lechin, F Central and plasma 5HT,vagal tone and airways [letter]. Trends Pharmacol Sci 2000;21:425

[58] Lechin, F, van der Dijs, B, Lechin, AE Severe asthma and plasma serotonin [letter]. Allergy 2002;57:258-259

[59] Lechin, F, van der Dijs, B, Lechin, AE. Tianeptine, plasma serotonin and pulmonary hypertension [letter]. Lancet 2003;361:87

[60] Cattaneo, MG, Codignola, A, Vicentini, LM, et al Nicotine stimulates a serotonergic autocrine loop in human small-cell lung carcinoma. Cancer Res 1993;53:5566-5568

[61] Krommaydas G, Gourgoulianis K, Raftopoulos V, Kotrotsiou E. Antidepressant and asthma treatment. Int J Pulmon Med 2005:Volume 6, Number 1.

[62] Sugihara H, Ishihara K,Nogughi H:Clinical experience with amitriptyline (tryptanol) in the treatment of bronchial asthma Annals of Allergy 1965 ;23:422-429

[63] Krommydas G, Gourgoulianis KI, Angelopoulos N, Kotrotsiou E, Raftopoulos V, Molyvdas P-A. Depression and pulmonary function in outpatients with asthma. Resp Med 2004;98:220-24

[64] Wright JR, Rodriguez M, Cohen S: Review of psychosocial stress and asthma: an intergrated biopsychosocial approach. Thorax 1998;53:1066 - 1074

[65] Krommydas G, Gourgoulianis KI, Karamitsos K, Krapis K, Molyvdas PA Therapeutic value of antidepressants in asthma. Med Hypotheses.2004 ;64:938-40

[66] Lechin F, van der Dijs B, Lechin AE.Treatment of bronchial asthma with Tianeptine. Methods Find Exp Clin Pharmacol.2004 ; 26 :1-5

[67] Fitzgerald J, Boulet L, Follows R. The CONCEPT trial: a 1-year, multicenter, randomized, double- blind, double dummy comparison of a stable dosing regimen of salmeterol/fluticasone propionate with an adjustable maintenance dosing regimen of formoterol/budesonide in adults with persistent asthma. Clinical Therapeutics 2005;27(4):393-406.

[68] Axelrod D, Bielory L. Fexofenadine hydrochloride in the treatment of allergic disease. J Asthma Allergy. 2008; 1: 19–29.

[69] Lee DKC, Catherine M. Jackson, Kay Haggart and Brian J. Lipworth. Repeated Dosing Effects of Mediator Antagonists in Inhaled Corticosteroid-Treated Atopic Asthmatic Patients. *Chest* 2004;125:1372-1377

[70] Docstoc. Depression and Asthma. www.docstoc.com/docs/48048960/Depression-and-Asthma

[71] Lomia M. Bronchial asthma as neurogenic inflammatory paroxysmal disease: mechanisms and therapy. http://www.asthma.ge/]

Section 2

Evidence-Based Strategies in Emergency Medicine

Chapter 4

Hypertensive Emergencies

Tomas Janota

Additional information is available at the end of the chapter

http://dx.doi.org/10.5772/59005

1. Introduction

The severest hypertensive states pose an immediate threat to life. To be able to manage these situations, physicians need well-defined recommendations; however, as with some other emergencies, only few evidence-based strategies have been developed to date.[1] As randomized, placebo-controlled trials are very difficult to design and conduct, most guidelines and recommendations are based just on experience. The recommendations and opinions in the present chapter draw mainly from national, European, and American guidelines for the treatment of hypertension, and on guidelines of professional societies such as the European Stroke Organisation as well as the experience gained in the author´s health-care center.[2-6]

2. Terminology

The terminology used for severe hypertensive states is not fully consistent, clear, and systematic. Severe hypertension-associated states can be divided into **hypertensive emergencies** and **hypertensive urgencies** under the general title **a hypertensive cris**is.

Hypertensive emergencies (HE) referring to more severe hypertensive states are defined as an acute, life-threatening states due to a sudden marked rise in blood pressure (BP) resulting in complaints and damage to the structure of some organs. [2-6] High BP leads to the development of acute problems and presentation of organ damage when reaching systolic and diastolic BP usually greater than 220 mm Hg and 120 mm Hg, respectively. However, in individuals so far normotensive, a hypertension may lead to a critical condition such as eclampsia already at a systolic BP of 170 mm Hg. The severity of the condition is dependent mainly on organ damage, not solely on the level of BP. The immediately threatened vital organs include the central nervous system and the cardiovascular system. Any damage to other organs (particularly the kidneys and eyes) is essentially always of primarily vascular etiology; hence, these organs are referred to as target ones. It is reasonable to refer to manifestation of damage since milder damage is often likely to go undetected. Importantly, damage to the central nervous and cardiovascular systems may pose an immediate threat to life. However, even manifestation of damage to another organ is associated with an increased risk of sudden damage to organs performing vital functions.[2-6]

According to the guidelines of the European Society of Hypertension (ESH) and the European Society of Cardiology (ESC), **hypertensive emergencies comprise**: hypertensive encephalopathy, hypertension with heart failure (including acute so-colled flash pulmonary oedema conditioned by sudden increase in BP), hypertension in acute coronary syndromes, hypertension in aortic dissection, hypertension in intracranial hemorrhage and ischemic stroke, sympathetic crises due to pheochromocytoma or an abuse of so-called recreational drugs (amphetamine, LSD, cocaine, ecstasy/MDMA etc.), perioperative hypertension, eclampsia/ severe pre-eclampsia and acute renal failure in hypertension (Table 1). Some listed HE are not accompanied by organ damage but the instability of the circulatory status and threats to the structure and function of organs belongs them between HE. In the European guidelines, the list of situations classified as HE is preceded by the word „primarily"[4]; hence the item is open for inclusion of other conditions. The current definition also seeks to avoid taking a clear position on the causality of hypertension and organ dysfunction as the degree of causality is frequently unclear.

Hypertensive ugencies should be characterized by complaints yet without manifest organ damage, with BP greater than 180/110 mmHg. These states include accelerated and malignant hypertension, postoperative hypertension, and hypertension in chronic heart failure. In addition to high BP (diastolic BP typically greater than 140 mm Hg), **accelerated hypertension** is characterized by vascular injury presenting with retinal hemorrhage and exudate formation. The **malignant hypertension** is more over associated with papilledema and/or renal injury and encephalopathy, manifestations of organ damage characteristic for HE. [2-6] From this perspective, it seems questionable resolution HE and hypertensive urgencies. The most recent joint ESH a ESC guidelines no longer list the term urgent hypertensive state as it usually does not require specific therapeutic strategies and hospitalization in the intensive care unit (ICU). Management of it is based on stepping up standard therapy with oral medications. Only in cases where it fails or in specific cases not allowing oral administration is parenteral treatment used.[4]

3. Etiology and prevalence of hypertensive emergencies

A role in the etiology of emergent hypertensive states is most often played by inadequate treatment of known hypertension and therapy discontinuation. [2,3,7] Pathophysiological mechanisms include a sudden rise in peripheral vascular resistance and systemic vasoconstriction due to activation of the renin-angiontension-aldosterone system, sympathoadrenal system, endothelin, exogenous factors, injury to the central nervous system, bleeding, tumor or ischemia, or perioperative stress. Except for conditions associated with renal failure, increased natriuresis and vasoconstriction result in reduced vascular filling. This can be effectively managed by afterload reduction; diuretic use is less effective. Hypertensive encephalopathy develops due to cerebral edema, which forms once the autoregulatory capacity of blood flow through brain arteries has been exceeded. The autoregulatory threshold is typically a mean BP of 140 mm Hg; however, the value may be higher in protracted severe hypertension. Other factors contributing to the development of edema include both hydrostatic mechanisms and changes in the vascular wall.[8]

The exact prevalence of severe hypertensive states is not known. These states occur more frequently in patients with nephrogenic hypertension and hyperaldosteronism. An emergent hypertensive status develops in about 1% of hypertensives during their lifetime.[9] An earlier US study reported about 8% and 16% of patients presenting at medical part of the emergency department with emergent and urgent hypertensive states, respectively.[10] In the experience of the author of this chapter, about 5% of patients admitted to the Intensive Cardiac Care Unit are diagnosed to have states somehow related to severe hypertension.

4. Clinical picture

The most frequent complaints accompanying HE include chest pain (27%), dyspnea (22%), headache (22%), epistaxis (17%), weakness and psychomotorical agitation (10%), whereas other authors list headache (49%) and weakness (22%) as the most frequently experienced problems.[5,8] Other complaints include palpitations, nausea, vomiting, anxiety and feeling of illness. Organ damage manifests itself most often as cerebral stroke (24%), lung edema (23%), neurological deficit (21%), and hypertensive encephalopathy (16%). Cerebral hemorrhage is diagnosed as little as 4.5% of cases (Tab. 2).[10] Retinal hemorrhage, exudates, and papilledema can also occur, indicating damage to other organs. These lesions do not subside until after several weeks since BP reduction. Oliguria, hyperazotemia, and proteinuria signal renal injury. Patients complaining of concomitant chest pain or other discomfort or with EKG-documented ST-segment depressions and a mild increase in cardiac troponins in serum can be diagnosed, according to the Universal definition of myocardial infarction, as type 2 myocardial infarction due to an imbalance between oxygen demand and supply.[11]

5. Examinations

Given the possibility of coarctation, atheorsclerosis of brachial arteries or, possibly, aortic dissection, BP should be measured on both arms. Measurement of BP in the lower limbs will rule out stenosis of arteries in both arms, a rare occurence. Blood pressure is measured using a properly-sized cuff to match the limb circumference. During subsequent managements in the ICU, BP is commonly measured noninvasively at intervals of 5 minutes to 1 hour depending on the severity of organ damage and BP level and instability. Only in cases of persisting instability of BP and its difficult control, or with conditions such as dissecting aneurysm requiring controlled hypotension, is it necessary to insert an arterial line. The cannula should be preferably inserted after a reduction of BP by initial therapy in some compressible brachial artery. An integral part of physical examination is neurological assessment to guide therapy. Basic biochemical tests including plasma concentration of minerals, urea, creatinine, markers of myocardial necrosis, natriuretic peptides, liver tests (to determine elimination of drugs), urinalysis (albuminuria, hematuria, crystaluria, etc.), and blood count should be done immediately. Additional examinations include EKG, chest x-ray, and fundoscopy. Echocardiography is performed in the context of hypertension primarily to assess the presence of myocardial dysfunction, muscle hypertrophy or, possibly, to roule out dissection of the aorta. Patient diagnosed to have focal neurological deficit and encephalopathy require a brain CT. Additional examinations are performed based on the patient´s current status.

6. Management

Management of HE should be instituted immediately and continued in ICU. Therapy during transportation to the ICU is of course limited espetially by the possibilities of BP measurement as well as by continuous dousing of IV medication.

The goal of treatment is to reduce BP and thus to prevent target organ damage and threat of life. However, very high BP must not be reduced very quickly. Too rapid and large BP reduction could be as dangerous and harmful as high BP. Blood pressure should be reduced by only 20-25% of baseline value over the first hours or until reaching levels 150-160/100-110 mm Hg. Alternatively, it is recommended to decrease mean BP to below 110-115 mm Hg within 30-60 minutes and, possibly, continue depending on the response and, most importantly, on how the patient tolerates the reduction. An abrupt fall in BP may-primarily in elderly patients with coronary and cerebrovascular atherosclerosis-impair organ perfusion, possibly resulting in acute renal failure, ischemic heart and cerebral events, renal artery occlusion and, eventually, acute blindness. However, in many cases, it is impossible to achieve a steady reduction of BP as recommended, particularly in settings where invasive monitoring is unavailable. A frequent occurrence is a rapid fall of an initially resistant high BP once contributing factors such as fear, uneasines and pain have disappeared. Achievement of the target BP for the chronic treatment is supposed within 1-2 days.[2-6]

The drugs to be used should have a short half-time of action but a rapid onset of action. They should be administered intravenously. When planning to use a combination of such agents, it is reasonable to have several venous access sites allowing for their separate administration. This often requires the insertion of a central venous line. Some agents such as nimodipine should only be administered via a central venous catheter. On the other hand, any inadvertent puncture of an artery in an effort to cannulate a central vein of a patient with poorly controlled high BP carries the risk of major bleeding.[2-6]

Hypertensive urgencies can usually be managed by intensification of their oral therapy or its complementation. Parenteral therapy is not started unless oral therapy has failed or is

http://dx.doi.org/10.5772/59005

not accepted. Stay at ICU is not necessary. According to US authors, therapy can even be administered on an outpatient basis with intensive patient monitoring over the first days of therapy. [2,10]

7. Drugs for IV therapy of severe hypertension

The agents currently available for parenteral therapy include nitrates, urapidil, diuretics, angiotensin-converting blockers, calcium-channel blockers, beta-blockers, alpha-blockers, combined alpha-and beta-blockers, clonidine and fenoldopam.(Tab. 3) [2,3,6]

Nitrates (isosorbide dinitrateand glycerol-trinitrate) can be the drugs of first choice in almost all conditions. They can be combined with most of the other hypertensive classes and are a reasonable option for pre-hospital initiation of therapy, with a rapid onset of effect within 2-5 minutes to subside within 5-10 minutes. Nitrates are applied as continuous infusion at a rate of 0.5-10 mg/h. At higher doses veno-as well as arteriodilation is present. If given at high doses, the antihypertensive effect is usually not incremental, yet the risk of headache is increased. As the patient becomes tolerant to continuous infusion, nitrates should be stopped discontinued after 2 days.[12] Sublingual nitrate administration may result in too rapid fall of BP; the effect is short-term, hence this use is not reasonable.

Sodium nitroprusside is one of the most effective drugs with an almost immediate onset of effect and a short half-life, with the BP reduction resolving within 2-3 minutes. Infusion therapy is started at 0.2 μg/ kg /min. The rate of infusion is every 3-5 minutes doubled to achieve the target BP. The speed of the application usually does not exceed 10 μg/kg/min. The mechanism of its action is vasodilation; however, unlike nitrates, it exerts a more marked effect on arterioles. As a major drawback of sodium nitroprusside is its photosensitivity. It should be infused via dark-color sets, with the infusion bottle covered with a light-tight material. Infusion at a higher rate for 2-3 days, particularly in patients with renal failure, is associated with the risk of intoxication with thiocyanate, a sodium nitroprusside metabolite, manifesting itself with confusion, nausea, and acidosis. Thiocyanate intoxication can be prevented by monitoring its levels. Concentration greater than 10 mg/100 ml is toxic. Alternatively, toxicity can be reduced by thiosulfate infusion, continuous infusion of 10% sodium thiosulfate in a volume ratio of 10:1 (nitroprusside : thiosulfate).[13]

Urapidil hydrochloride is an antagonist of peripheral alpha1-postsynaptic receptors; animal studies have shown it is also an antagonist of central 5-hydroxytryptamine-1A receptors. It has been shown to decrease particularly peripheral vascular resistance withe the resultant decreas both preload and afterload. It has been associated with marked selective renal and pulmonary vasodilation. Unlike other vasodilators, it does not induce appreciable tachycardia, likely due to central modulation of cardiovascular centers via 5-hydroxytryptamin receptores. Its other effects include mild β1-blockade. Urapidil decreases systolic and diastolic BP in a balanced manner. The onset of its effect is virtually immediate, peaking within 2-5 minutes. Its antihypertensive effect subsides completely within 4 hours at most. Regarding its use in stroke, it should be noted that, unlike other antihypertensives, urapidil does not exacerbate cerebral edema and intracranial pressure. Urapidil is extensively metabolized (50-70%) in the liver, with 15-50 % of the drug excreted through the kidneys. Side effects are rather rare and mild. The most frequent ones include tachycardia, sweating, chest discomfort, dyspnea, and weakness. If given at higher doses, urapidil has a sedative action. Literary data suggest that its antihypertensive effect is similar to that of enalaprilat, nitroprusside, nifedipine, and dihydralazine. Resistance to urapidil occurs more rarely with with enalaprilate and nifedipine. As a standard policy, therapy with urapidil is initiated with a bolus followed immediately by continuous infusion. It is recommended to give a 10-50 mg bolus over 20 seconds depending on the BP level and clinical status. If there is a sufficient decrease in BP within 5 minutes of bolus administration, continuous therapy can be initiated. In the event of an inadequate effect of the first bolus, especially when rapid BP control is needed, additional boluses should be administered with patient status to be re-assessed at a 5-minute interval. While repeat bolus administration until achieving target BP with subsequent maintenance therapy provide for the quickest BP normalization, the total dose of initial boluses should preferably not exceed 50 mg because of the risk of a sudden severe fall of BP. A dose of 100 mg is only an alternative for very severe resistant hypertension with signs of organ damage. By contrast, in patients raising concern of a major fall in BP and a less emergent status, therapy can be initiated directly with continuous i.v. infusion at a rate of 120 mg/h without initial bolus administration with a subsequent decrease in the infusion rate once the BP has decreased. It is recommended to continue with maintenance therapy at a rate of 2–10 mg/h depending on the patient´s status and their BP level. The maximum recommended rate for long-term administration is 30 mg/h. The maximum recommended therapy duration 7 days based primarily on toxicology studies not exceeding the above period of time. Longer administration requires closer monitoring of the patient´s status. In the presence of liver or renal failure, it is also recommended only to perform closer hemodynamic monitoring without dose reduction. Given the risk of severe hypotension, combinations of urapidil with another alpha-blocker are contraindicated. Overdose with urapidil or development of side effects can usually be simply managed by dose reduction or therapy discontinuation. In persistent moderate hypotension, the procedure of choice is, of course, volume expansion or, possibly, IV catecholamine administration.

In the case of perioperative hypertension, the recommendation is to initiate therapy with a 25 mg bolus; if effective within 2 minutes of the initial bolus, the patient can be switched to maintenance therapy. The recommended dose of urapidil for maintenance perioperative therapy is 60-180 mg/hour. No data regarding gestational hypertension and urapidil excretion to breast milk are currently available.[14-19]

As urapidil has not yet been approved by the US Food and Drug Administration (FDA), it is simply not mentioned in a number of texts published in the USA.

Clonidine is a centrally-acting drug. It acts primarily via alpha2-receptors to produce protracted vasodilation. Its plasma half-life is in the range of 12 hours. Clonidine could be administered IV as a very slow 150 μg bolus (over 10-15 minutes) or infusion at rate 1-2 μg/kg/min. Maximal daily dose is 750 μg. At present, its use is reserved for combinations in resistant hypertension and situations requiring sedative effect. Because of the risk of potential respiratory center inhibition, it can be used with advantage in patients with mechanical ventilation.[20,21]

Fenoldopam mesylate is a **selective D1 dopamin receptor agonist** with a half-time of elimination as short as 5 minutes. It causes renal, mesenteric, and coronary arteriodilation while also increasing sodium excretion. Hypotensive efficacy is similar to that of sodium nitroprusside. As a side effect, it produces a tendency to developing tachycardia. However, its co-administration with betablockers may be extremely harmful. Usual initial dosage is 0.1–0.3 μg/kg/min. To achieve desired therapeutic effect, may titrate dosage upward or downward in increments of 0.05–0.1 μg /kg/min.[22,23]

Furosemide is a **diuretic** suitable for emergent situations. Needless to say, its use is appropriate in heart failure and conditions associated with edema formation. As a drug of first choice it is little effective. Ahigh BP induces natriuresis, which, together with frequently concomitant nausea/vomiting, results in fluid depletion and need for hydration rather than diuretic use. Not infrequently is BP reduction seen following saline administration.

Enalaprilate is the only **angiotensin-converting enzyme** available in injectable form. Its major advantage is its favorable effect on cerebral vascular autoregulation. When administered i.v., its onset of action occurs within 15 minutes, with its peak effect expected after 1-4 hours. Regrettably, the strength and duration of its action are variable lasting as it may 6 but, also 24 hours. Enaprilate is excreted via the kidney. Its dose should be adjusted in patients with renal insufficiency. Contraindications to enaprilate use are identical with those applicable to other angiotensin-converting enzyme inhibitors. As a result, enaprilate is used mostly as a drug of second or third choice in resistant hypertension on the assumption it will not induce undesirable hypotension. The risk of hypotension is particularly high in patients experiencing dehydration. Enalapril is administered as a 0.625 to 1.25 mg bolus, most often at a 6-hour interval depending on the effect. The body of experience with continuous administration is fairly limited.[24]

In outpatient practice, and as a **first-aid measure**, crushing of a tablet of the short-acting angiotensin-converting enzyme inhibitor captopril at a dose of 25-50 mg may occasionally be helpful. However, in really serious situations with uncertainty regarding future course including the state of consciousness, oral captopril should not be administered.

Calcium-channel blockers have proved effective, particularly in the management and prevention of vasopasms in subarachnoidal hemorrhage. By contrast, concerns have been voiced about their use in ischemic stroke where they may exacerbate collateral cerebral edema. Favorable experience has been obtained with the dihydropyridine-type drugs **nicardipine** and **nimodipine**. A drawback of nimodipine is has to be infused via a central venous catheter. Usual infusion rate is 0.5-2.0 mg/h. It is used preferably only in cases of subarachnoidal hemorrhage indicated for neurosurgery. In the event of surgical intervention during treatment, administration of nimodipine should be continued for at least five days. [25] Currently the most promising agent is the novel ultrashort-acting agent **clevidipine** inducing selective arteriolar dilation including the coronary bed, with onset of action occurring within 2-4 minutes and lasting 5-15 minutes. Dose range between 2 and 16 mg/h. Like nitroprusside or calcium-channel blockers clevidipine produce a marked decrease in BP with a mild rise in heart rate and cardiac output. Clevidipine provided in the study ECLIPSE better blood pressure control compared to nitroglycerine and nitroprusside.[26-28] Less experience in emergent hypertensive stats is available with continuous administration of **verapamil** slowing down heart rate and exerting a somewhat negative inotropic effect. Its use has been suggested in hypertensive states associated with tachycardia at total dose up to 100 mg/day.[29]

Betablockers are the drugs of choice in hypertension and tachycardia. They are particularly advantageous in combination with urapidil or nitroprusside. Betablockers are one of the few classes of drugs appropriate for use in patients with severe hypertension and ischemic stroke. They are traditionally used in the treatment of dissecting aneurysms as they are believed to reduce pulse pressure thereby decreasing aortic wall stress; however, their effect on Dp/Dt has been recently challenged. Betablockers are recommended for use in intraoperative hypertension. Particularly **esmolol**, highly beta1-selective and ultra-short acting drug with peak effect after administration of 500 mg/kg bolus followed by continuous i.v. administration reached during 5 minutes and resolving within 10-30 minutes is recommended in HE. The dose is up-titrated at a 5-minute interval with or without boluses. Continuous dose range between 25 and 300 μg/kg/min. [30] **Metoprolol** in continuous infusion at a rate 1-5 mg/h could be also effective but with longer hilf-time and lower selectivity compare to esmolol. Boluses of 2.5-5 mg administered one to three times as needed to achieve goal are also frequently used.[31]

Labetalol is both a selective alpha1-blocker and predominantly a non-selective beta-blocker. Treatment is initiated depending on its effect with 5-160 mg boluses administered repeatedly at 2-10 minutes to a maximum dose of 300 mg. Labetalol can also be administered continuously at a rate 2 mg/minutes up to a total dose of 300 mg/24 hours. The effect sets in within 5-10 minutes and resolves within 2-6 hours. A traditional indication-apparently based, in particular, on the absence of adverse experience-is management of pre-eclampsia/eclampsia. It is also the drug of choice in other situations, except those contraindicated to beta-blocker use.[32] In the USA, labetalol is the drug most often used in the treatment of HE.

Alpha-blockerphentolamine is indicated espetially for the control of hypertensive episodes that may occur in a patient with pheochromocytoma as a result of stress or manipulation during preoperative preparation and surgical excision. Boluse dose of 5 mg should be applied fast with BP measurements in 1 minute's intervals during first minutes after administration. Repeated administration could be necessary during surgery.[33]

8. Management in specific situations

The choice of individual classes of drugs depends on the underlying disease resulting in HE or it is associated with. To date, only few randomized studies have been conducted evaluating treatment of HE and almost no studies designed for head-to-head comparison of various drugs.[1]

Ischemic stroke usually results in an increase in BP for 1-4 days. Drug therapy of this type of hypertension is associated with the risk of impairing vascular autoregulation with a subsequent decrease in blood flow in the vicinity of the ischemic focus.[35,36] Besides, patients are also increasingly susceptible to an abrupt fall in BP. The benefit of BP reduction in the acute stroke has not been documented except for situations with a diastolic BP > 130 mm Hg conclusively associated with progressive damage to brain structures. It is recommended not to decrease BP until it levels rise above 200-210/120 mmHg. Within the first hours after hospitalisation, BP should be decreased by 10% of the baseline value. The target BP is below 180/105 mmHg. As BP increases, the risk of secondary bleeding is also likely to increase, apparently not a rare occurrence even without marked hypertension. In patients indicated for thrombolytic therapy it is recommended to reduce BP below 180/110 mm Hg.[35,36] Substantial reduction in BP may be indicated only by the simultaneous occurrence of diseases such as heart failure, acute coronary syndrome or aortic dissection. Fast but short acting i.v. drugs are preferred for the accurate titration of the effect. Drugs with side effect of steal phenomenon, worsening of brain oedema due to brain vasodilator effect are to be excluded. The treatment is recommended especially with medication such as labetalol and betablockers. A good experience is with fast and realtively shortly acting urapidil inspite of the risks of the central sedative effect. Enalaprilat may have a beneficial effect on cerebral vascular autoregulation but it is associated with the risk of inducing undesirable protracted hypotension.

In **hemorrhagic stroke**, the recommendation is to reduce BP already at levels 160/110 mm Hg, with target BP being 140-160/90 mm Hg.[1] No additional BP correction is necessary once bleeding has been controlled. In the presence of vasospasms, the target BP level is 180-220 mm Hg once bleeding has been controlled. The drugs used in hemorrhagic stroke are the same as those indicted for ischemic stroke Moreover dihydropyridine calcium-channel blockers can also be used for continuous i.v. therapy, particularly in subarachnoidal hemorrage. Even in the absence of elevated BP, calcium-channel blockers can prevent the development of vasospams, a frequent occurrence in subarachnoidal hemorrhage.[37]

In **hypertensive encephalopathy**, therapy can be initiated with a nitrate. Other recommended agents include parenteral labetalol, esmolol, and enalaprilate. When administering higher doses of urapidil, one should be aware of its sedative effect carrying the risk of impaired consciousness. High BP reduction results in a prompt resolution of symptoms such as confusion, sleepiness to comatose states, seizures or focal and sensory disorders. A typical up to diagnostic feature of hypertensive encephalopathy is the disappearance of impaired consciousness after diastolic BP reduction below 100-110 mm Hg. However, it is always critical to exclude another organic cause of symptoms attributed to hypertensive encephalopathy.[2,6]

In **congestive heart failure**, treatment is initiated with nitrates and diuretics. The drug of choice is enalaprilate or, alternatively, urapidil decreasing, in a desirable manner, simultaneously preload and afterload. In this context, fenoldopam seems to be a most promising drug. An important part of therapy is sedation. In heart failure, BP should be reduced more aggressively to levels below 140/90 mm Hg.

Acute coronary syndromes in hypertension are managed with parenteral nitrates combined with betablockers or, possibly, with urapidil. A critical consideration in these conditions are sedation and pain relief. This therapy should precede more aggressive antihypertensive therapy as a high BP is most often due to pain and anxiety. On the other hand, BP normalization may contribute to reduction of myocardial load and pain relief.

Acute aortic dissection requires reduction of systolic BP to 100 mm Hg within 20 minutes, most often using a combination of a nitrate, nitroprusside or urapidil with a betablocker. Even when dissection is only suspected, systolic BP should be lowered to 120 mm Hg within 20 minutes. [2,6]

In **acute renal failure** with severe hypertension, the most effective drugs include urapidil, nitropruside, clonidine, and fenoldopam.[2,6,38] In the presence of hyperhydratio, extracorporeal elimination can be indicated in addition to high-dose furosemide. Aggressive therapy should be initiated particularly in the presence of a sudden rise of azotemia and so-called shadows of damaged red blood cells in the urine and dysmorphous red blood cells in urinalysis in phase contrast imaging. A steady BP reduction is especially important in renal injury.

In **pheochromocytome** with severe hypertension, an advantageous approach is to initiate therapy with an isosorbide dinitrate-type nitrate. In more severe states, treatment is based on a combination of urapidil with a betablocker. Given its predominantly betablocking action, extra caution should be exercised when using labetalol. The alphablocker phentolamine is employed primarily in surgical removal of pheochromocytoma. [2,6]

Treatment of **hypertension induced by amphetamine or cocaine abuse** is guided by principles similar to those with pheochromocyte. Excessive release of catecholamines has also been reported. [2,6]

Hypertension induced by other exogenous substances is likely to be associated with vasoconstriction and tachycardia, which is why appropriate therapy includes vasodilatators and drugs with bradycardiac activity. [2,6]

In **eclampsia/severe pre-eclampsia**, treatment should be started already at BP > 170/110 mm Hg. Labetalol is the traditionally recommended drug. As with a variety of other conditions, treatment can be initiated with a nitrate switching the patient to urapidil with a betablocker in resistant hypertension. Nitroprusside can only be administrated over a short period time. While the effect of verapamil can also be tested but the drug should not be administered with MgSO4 commonly given in eclampsia because of the risk of aggregation.[2,6]

In **intra-operative hypertension**, the preferred drug is the ultrashort-acting betablocker esmolol. The drugs of choice include nitrates, urapidil, and dihydropyridine-type calcium-channel blockers. [2,6]

A switchover from parenteral to oral therapy should be undertaken once the patient has stabilized to make hospitalization as short as possible. It is reasonable to test the efficacy of the chosen medication for at least 1-3 days in the hospital setting. After discharge, the patient should be followed-up at intervals ranging from one week to several weeks.

http://dx.doi.org/10.5772/59005

9. Prognosis

Uncontrolled malignant hypertension results in 90% one-year mortality due to heart failure, stroke, or renal failure. There are virtually no data from randomized controlled studies showing how treatment with individual drugs affects mortality and morbidity, and whether any drug is superior to another one. Introduction of novel ultrashort-acting and well tolerated drug are expected to provide the greatest benefit in the near future.

Hypertensive encephalopathy
Hypertension with heart failure
Hypertension in acute coronary syndromes
Hypertension in aortic dissection
Hypertension in intracranial hemorrhage
Hypertension in ischemic stroke
Sympathetic crises due to pheochromocytoma
Sympathetic crises after abuse of so-called recreational drugs (amphetamine, LSD, cocaine, ecstasy/MDMA)
Perioperave hypertension
Eclampsia and severe pre-eclampsia
Acute renal failure in hypertension

Table 1. Hypertensive emergencies

Complaints	%
Chest pain	27
Dyspnea	22
Headache	22-40
Nosebleed	17
Weakness and psychomotor agitation	10-22
Organ damage	
Increase in troponin levels above the diagnostic cut-off for AMI (Type-2 AMI)	38
Stroke	24
Pulmonary edema	23
Neurological deficit	21

Complaints	%
Hypertensive encephalopathy	16
Cerebral hemorrhage	4.5

Table 2. Most common manifestations of emergent and urgent hypertensive states

Nitrates (isosorbid-dinitrate, glycerol-trinitrate) Mechanism of action: venodilatation, at higher doses arteriodilation Onset of action: maximal effect within 2-5 minutes Duration of action: 5-10 minutes Specific indications: medication of choice in almost all situations, mostly first choice medication, advantageous especially for heart failure and acute coronary syndromes Specific contraindications: ischemic stroke
Sodium nitroprusside Mechanism of action: arterio- as well as venodilation Onset of action: almost immediate, maximal effect within 2-3 minutes Duration of action: minutes, circulatory half-life about 2 minutes Specific indications: particularly resistant hypertension, controlled hypotension Specific contraindications: liver failure, severe cardiovascular stenotic defects, ischemic stroke
Urapidil hydrochloride Mechanism of action: vasodilatation (antagonist of peripheral alpha1-postsynaptic receptors, antagonist of central 5-hydroxytryptamine-1A receptors), mild beta1-blockade Onset of action: almost immediate, maximal effect within 2-5 minutes Duration of action: up to 4 hours Specific indications: sever and resistant hypertension in almost all situations, controlled hypotension Specific contraindications: no data regarding lactation
Clonidine Mechanism of action: vasodilatation (centrally acting alpha2-agonist), sedative, analgesic and opioid properties Onset of action: almost immediate Duration of action: plasma half-life is ranging between 10 and 20 hours Specific indications: for combinations in resistant hypertension and situations requiring sedative effect Specific contraindications: severe brady-arrhythmias resulting from either sick sinus syndrome or AV block of 2nd or 3rd degree

http://dx.doi.org/10.5772/59005

Fenoldopam mesylate

Mechanism of action: selective renal dopamine D1 receptor agonist; renal, mesenteric and coronary arteriodilation, increase of sodium excretion

Onset of action: rapid, most of the antihypertensive effect attained in 15 minutes

Duration of action: quickly reversible, half-life 5-10 minutes

Specific indications: particularly useful in patients with severe hypertension associated with end-organ renal damage or volume overload

Specific contraindications: administration with beta-blockers

Enalaprilate

Mechanisms of action: angiotensin-converting enzyme, normalization of cerebral vascular autoregulation

Onset of action: within 15 minutes, peak effect after 1-4 hours

Duration of action: 6 - 24 hours

Specific indications: drug of two to third choice in resistant hypertension

Specific contraindication: pregnancy, common contraindications to angiotensin-converting enzyme inhibitors

Nimodipine

Mechanisms of action: calcium-channel blocker with preferential activity on cerebral vessels; increase of cerebral perfusion, particularly in poorly perfused areas, by arterial dilatation

Onset of action: almost immediate

Duration of action: the half-life is 1.1 - 1.7 hours, the terminal half-life is 5-10 hours

Specific indications: preferably aneurysmal subarachnoidal hemorrhage

Specific contraindication: lack of a central venous catheter

Clevidipin

Mechanisms of action: calcium-channel blocker; selective arteriolodilatation including coronary arteries

Onset of action: within 2–4 min.

Duration of action: 5–15 min.

Specific indications: rapid reduction of BP in the perioperative setting

Specific contraindication: must not be used in patients with defective lipid metabolism accompanied by hyperlipidemia.

Verapamil

Mechanisms of action: calcium-channel blocker; decrease in peripheral vascular resistance, without an increase in heart rate as a reflex response

Onset of action: within 5 min.

Duration of action: half-life between 3.5 and 7.4 hours

Specific indications: hypertension with tachycardia and contraindications to beta-blockers

Specific contraindication: common to calcium-channel blockers	
Esmolol	
Mechanisms of action: beta1-selective blocker	
Onset of action: maximal effect of the selected dose within 5 min. after bolus	
Duration of action: 10-30 min., half-life 9 min.	
Specific indications: perioperative hypertension, aortic dissection, ischemic stroke, acute coronary syndrome	
Specific contraindication: pregnancy, common contraindications to beta-blockers	
Metoprolol	
Mechanisms of action: selective beta-blocker	
Onset of action: within 5 min.	
Duration of action: to 4 hours, elimination half-life 1-9 hours, average 3.5 hours	
Specific indications: aortic dissection, acute coronary syndrome	
Specific contraindication: pregnancy, common contraindications to beta-blockers	
Labetalol	
Mechanisms of action: non-selective beta-blocker, weak alpha-blocker	
Onset of action: within 5-10 min.	
Duration of action: 2-6 hours	
Specific indications: eclampsia, any severe hypertension	
Specific contraindication: common contraindications to beta-blockers	
Phentolamine	
Mechanisms of action: non-selective alpha-blocker	
Onset of action: minutes	
Duration of action: 2-4 hours	
Specific indications: during surgical manipulation with phaeochromocytoma	
Specific contraindication: common contraindications to alpha-blockers	

Table 3. Medication for the management of hypertensive emergencies

Author details

Tomas Janota*

Address all correspondence to: tomas.janota@vfn.cz

Cardio ICU, 3rd Department of Internal Medicine, Všeobecná fakultní nemocnice(University Hospital), Prague, Czech Republic

References

[1] Perez MI, Musini VM. Pharmacological interventions for hypertensive emergencies: a Cochrane systematic review. J Hum Hypertens 2008; 22: 596–607

[2] Elliott WJ. Clinical features in the management of selected hypertensive emergencies. Prog Cardiovasc Dis. 48: 2006; 316-325

[3] Hypertensive emergency and urgency. Herz 2004 ;29: 354

[4] The Task Force for the Management of Arterial Hypertension of the European Society of Hypertension and of the European Society of Cardiology. Guidelines Committee. 2007 Guidelines for the Management of Arterial Hypertension. J Hypertens 2007; 25: 1105-1187

[5] Joint National Committee on Prevention, Detection, Evaluation, and Treatment of High Blood Pressure. National Heart, Lung, and Blood Institute; National High Blood Pressure Education Program Coordinating Committee: Seventh Report of the Joint National Committee on Prevention, Detection, Evaluation, and the Treatment of High Blood Pressure. Hypertension. 42: 2003; 1206-1252

[6] Janota T. Akutní hypertenzní stavy a jejich terapie Cor Vasa 2011;53,8–9

[7] Bender SR, Fong MW, Heitz S, Bisognano JD. Characteristics and management of patients presenting to the emergency department with hypertensive urgency. J Clin Hypertens. 8: 2006; 12-18

[8] Gardner CJ, Lee K. Hypoperfusion syndrome: Insight into the Pathophysiology and Treatment of Hypertensive Encephalopathy. CNS Spectr 2007; 12: 35–42

[9] Slama M, Modeliar SS. Hypertension in the intensive care unit. Curr Opin Kardiol 2006; 21: 279-287

[10] Zampaglione B, Pascale C, Marchisio M, Cavallo-Perin P. Hypertensive urgencies and emergencies: Prevalence and clinical presentation. Hypertension. 27: 1996; 144-147

[11] K. Thygesen, J.S. Albert, H.D. White, et al.: The Writing Group on behalf of the Joint ESC/ACCF/AHA/WHF Task Force for the Universal Definition of Myocardial Infarction. Third universal definition of myocardial infarction European Heart Journal 33 (2012) 2551-2567.

[12] Isoket.spc.https://www.medicines.org.uk/emc/medicine/1887

[13] Nitroprusside.spc.http://www.medicines.org.uk/emc/medicine/651

[14] Schoetensack W, Bruckschen EG, Zech K. Urapidil. New Drugs Annual: Cardiovascular Drugs. 1983, 19

[15] Ramage AG. Influence of 5-HT1A receptor agonists on sympathetic and parasympathetic nerve activity. J Cardiovasc Pharmacol 1990; 15: S75–S85

[16] Verberne AJM, Rand MJ. Effect of urapidil on β-adrenoceptors of rat atria". Eur J Pharmacol 1985; 108: 193–196.

[17] Dooley M, Goa KL. Drugs. Urapidil. A reappraisal of its use in the management of hypertension.1998;56:929-955

[18] Wacker J, Werner P, Walter-Sack I, Bastert G. Treatment of hypertension in patients with pre-eclampsia: a prospective parallel-group study comparing dihydralazine with urapidil. Nephrol Dial Transplant. 1998;13,318-325

[19] Ebrantil.spc.http://db.cbg-meb.nl/Pars/h101891.pdf

[20] Hall et al. Sedative, analgesic and cognitive effects of clonidine infusions in humans. British Journal of Anaesthesia 2001;86:5-11

[21] Catapres.spc.http://www.medicines.org.uk/emc/medicine/283

[22] Murphy MB, Murray C, Shorten GD. Fenoldopam-a selective peripheral dopamine-receptor agonist for the treatment of severe hypertension. N Engl J Med. 2001; 345:1548-57

[23] Fenves AZ, Ram CV. Drug treatment of hypertensive urgencies and emergencies. Semin Nephrol. 25: 2005; 272-280

[24] DiPette DJ et al. Enalaprilat, an intravenous angiotensinconvertingenzyme inhibitor, inhypertensive crises Clin Pharmacol Therap 1985; 2: 199-204

[25] Dilceren.spc. http://www.medicines.org.uk/emc/medicine/5581

[26] Clevidipine.spc.http://www.medicines.org.uk/emc/medicine/5581

[27] Phung OJ, Baker WL, White CM et al. Clevidipine: An intravenous dihydropyridine calcium-channel blocker for the treatment of acute hypertension. Formulary 2009;44:102–107

[28] Cleviprex.spc.http://www.medicines.org.uk/emc/medicine/28128

[29] Isoptin.spc.http://www.medicines.ie/medicine/11962/SPC/

[30] Esmocard.spc.http://db.cbg-meb.nl/mri/spc/nlh-0779-002. pdf

[31] Betaloc.spc.http://www.medicines.org.uk/emc/medicine/152

[32] Trandate.spc.https://www.medicines.org.uk/emc/medicine/4297

[33] Regitin.http://www.old.health.gov.il/units/pharmacy/trufot/ alonim/4502.pdf

[34] Varon J. Diagnosis and management of labile blood pressure during acute cerebrovascular accidents and other hypertensive crises. Am J Emerg Med 2007; 25: 949–995

http://dx.doi.org/10.5772/59005

[35] European Stroke Initiative: European Stroke Initiative recommendations for stroke management. European Stroke Council, European Neurological Society and European Federation of Neurological Societies. Cerebrovasc Dis 2000;10:335-351

[36] The European Stroke Initiative Executive Committee and the EUSI Writing Committee: European Stroke Initiative Recommendations for Stroke Management – Update 2003. Cerebrovascular Disease 2003;16:311-337

[37] Steiner T, Kaste M, Forsting M, Mendelow D, Kwiecinski H, Szikora I, Juvela S, Marchel A, Chapot R, Cognard C, Unterberg A, Hacke W: Recommendations for the management of intracranial haemorrhage-part I: spontaneous intracerebral haemorrhage. The European Stroke Initiative Writing Committee and the Writing Committee for the EUSI Executive Committee. Cerebrovasc Disease 2006;22:294-316

[38] Devlin JW, Seta ML, Kanji S, Somerville AL. Fenoldopam versus nitroprusside for the treatment of hypertensive emergency. Ann Pharmacother. 38: 2004; 755-759

Section 3

New Approach In Management of Psychiatric Disorders

Chapter 5

Rational Polypharmacy in Psychiatry

S. Haque Nizamie and Sai Krishna Tikka

Additional information is available at the end of the chapter

http://dx.doi.org/10.5772/59004

1. Introduction

Dimensional approach in clinical psychopharmacology conceptualizes a disorder under multiple dimensions that are affected at a particular time. Impairments in multiple domains is a major factor leading to the fact that significant proportion of patients with various major psychiatric disorders does not achieve remission (McEvoy et al., 2006; Perlis et al., 2006; Rush et al., 2006). This model proposes to tackle each dimension independently as the interaction between the various dimensions remains to be accurately understood (Baruch et al., 1992). Such an approach has lead to use of several molecules in the treatment of a single condition, a situation that we often refer to as polypharmacy. Increasing frequency of polypharmacy (Mojtabai and Olfson, 2010) suggests that the major approach in pharmacological treatment of psychiatric disorders is the dimensional one.

Psychiatry being one of the most complex specialties among medicine, psychiatric diagnosis is based on subjective personal history and specifically constructed clinical criteria. There is a certain lack of empirical data and more so for objective laboratory tests. Moreover, with the increasing identification of comorbid conditions and evidence-based guidelines recommending an array of molecules in the treatment of a single disorder, without the emphasis on, preference has escalated the strategy of polypharmacy. The reported overall prevalence rates of polypharmacy in psychiatry vary between 13% to an alluring 90% (Kukreja et al., 2013).

2. Definition and classification

Although the term polypharmacy has been in use and has evolved for a very long time, a proper definition is still lacking. Majority of studies in psychiatry have used the criteria of "2 or more medications of the same chemical class or with the same or similar pharmacological actions to treat the same condition" (Kukreja et al., 2013). Apart from a trendy yet justifiable classification of polypharmacy into-"The Good, the Bad, and the Ugly" (Kingsbury and Lotito, 2007), several other classifications have been proposed to describe various types of polypharmacy (Table 1). Multiclass Polypharmacy is the most common type with prevalence of 20.9% among which combination of SSRI with a benzodiazepine is the most common. In the same class polypharmacy, treatment with several benzodiazepines is the most common (De las Cuevas and Sanz, 2004).

The basis for these classifications is discrete and hence there would be significant overlap when considering them together i.e. combination of lithium and fluoxetine in treating resistant depression is an example of therapeutic, multiclass, minor and rational polypharmacy. As positive outcome is the foundation for evidence based treatment, contra-therapeutic and rational polypharmacy are mutually exclusive. However, with wide inter-individual heterogeneity, one may consider none of the classes to be exclusively inseparable i.e. rational strategy of clozapine augmentation with olanzapine might result in worsening of metabolic status, resulting in contra-therapeutic polypharmacy.

Sl.no	Classification	Basis	Proposed by
1	• Therapeutic • Contra-therapeutic	Outcome	Werder and Preskorn, 2003
2	• Same class • Multiclass • Adjunctive • Augmentative • Total	Pharmacological class and appropriateness	National Association of State Mental Health Program Directors, 2001
3	• Minor • Moderate • Major	Number of drugs	Veehof et al., 2000
4	• Rational • Irrational	Rationality/ evidence base	Kingsbury et al., 2001

Table 1. Polypharmacy-several classifications

This narrative review considers various rational polypharmacy strategies in treating psychiatric disorders. Evidence base for polypharmacy strategies in individual disorders is highlighted with an emphasis on special settings.

3. Depression

Polypharmacy in the treatment of depression has an increasing trend. While 3.3% of depression patients received 3 or more drugs in 1970s, in 1990s the rate increased to 43.8% in an NIMH hospital (Frye et al., 2000). Although the exact share of rational polypharmacy could not be ascertained, evidence base for polypharmacy in depression management is satisfactory.

With a number of molecules with different mechanisms of action available, combination of any two compounds has a potential for an impressive strategy to treat depression that does not respond to antidepressant monotherapy (Moret, 2005). Combinations of certain antidepressants-mirtazapine combined with venlafaxine, fluoxetine and bupropion (in the order of highest response) have been shown to have better response rate than anti depressant monotherapy (fluoxetine plus placebo) (Blier et al., 2010). Blier and colleagues had also found that a combination of mirtazapine and paroxetine showed significantly higher response rates than either drug alone (Blier et al., 2009). There has been another study (Carpenter et al., 2002) that studied a selective serotonin reuptake inhibitor (SSRI) combined with mirtazapine and found the combination to be better. Nelson et al. (2004) found a combination of fluoxetine and desipramine to be better than either drug alone. Recently, Sung et al. (2012) compared escitalopram monotherapy with bupropion+escilatoplram and velnafaxine+mirtazapine and found that there was no significant difference in the adverse effect profile in both chronic and non chronic depression patients. However, they found no significant difference in either response or remission rates between the different treatment groups. Positive data from controlled trials on antidepressant combinations are restricted to mirtazapine as the combination drug questioning the generalizability of the findings to other combinations. Also these trials are not free of limitations: insufficient duration, lower doses of monotherapy agents, etc. (Rush, 2010). Trials including other agents like SAM (S-adenosyl-l-methionine) are not randomized controlled (Alpert et al., 2004).

Various augmentation drugs used in the treatment of depression in combination with an antidepressant are-atypical antipsychotics, lithium, hormonal drugs like thyroxine, estrogen and mifepristone, 5HT1A antagonists like pindolol, buspirone, and, stimulants like methylphenidate. Augmentation with atypical antipsychotics has been shown to be significantly more effective than placebo for response and remission. Although aripiprazole is the first pharmacologic agent of any type to be approved by the U.S. FDA for use as an augmentation agent in major depressive disorder, other agents have also been used. Among atypical antipsychotics, evidence is available for olanzapine in combination with fluoxetine, quetiapine and aripiprazole in combination with either SSRI or an SNRI and risperidone with various antidepressants (Nelson and Papakostas, 2009). While the meta-Analysis by Nelson and Papakostas (2009) conclude no significant differences in efficacy among the different agents, Connolly and Thase (2011) in their review give a preference to quetiapine and aripiprazole. Bauer et al. (2010) in their meta-analysis found significantly greater mean response rate in the lithium group than the placebo group. Apart from stating augmentation of antidepressants with lithium as the best-evidenced augmentation therapy in the treatment of depression, they also suggested a predictive role of the –50T/C single nucleotide polymorphism of the GSK3-beta gene (Bauer et al., 2010). However, Connolly and Thase (2011) question its generalizability stating lithium is only effective for use in combination with tricyclic antidepressants (TCAs) and that these trials included less treatment-resistant subjects than those who typically receive TCAs in current clinical settings. Triiodothyronine augmentation seems to offer better benefit/risk ratio for augmentation of modern antidepressants (Connolly and Thase, 2011). While trials on pindolol have failed to replicate positive effects, there is no clear consensus of the role of buspirone, mifepristone and methylphenidate (Moret, 2005). Although estrogen augmentation is effective, the response seems to be more restricted to menopausal women (Liu et al., 2004).

Surprisingly however, data from trials on combination of conventional antidepressants like tricyclic agents and MAO inhibitors or augmentation with first generation antipsychotics is sparse.

4. Bipolar disorder

4.1. Acute mania

In reality, less than 10% of acutely manic patients receive monotherapy. Clinical routine appears to be based on polypharmacy in bipolar patients (Peh and Tay 2008). In line with this clinical practice, RCT's suggest that addition of an antipsychotic to patients with persistent manic symptoms despite treatment with lithium or valproate has shown greater rates of acute efficacy than has continuation of lithium or valproate alone (Vieta et al., 2008). As to the important clinical question whether de novo combinations are better, there is very limited data. A greater efficacy of combination treatment is also supported by a meta-analysis of Smith et al. (2007) which showed that significantly more participants on co-therapy met the response criterion reductions. Such effects were demonstrated for haloperidol, olanzapine, risperidone and quetiapine when administered as co-therapy compared with monotherapy with lithium or valproate. Taken together, there is not enough unambiguous evidence that supports combination therapy as a general first line treatment (Grunze et al., 2009).

4.2. Acute bipolar depression

In the case of acute bipolar depression, the categories of evidence and grades of recommendation for pharmacological treatment are mentioned in table 2. Olanzapine+fluoxetine (Tohen et al. 2003; Brown et al. 2009), Lamotrigine+Lithium (van der Loos et al. 2009), Modafinil +ongoing treatment (Frye et al. 2007) and N-acetylcysteine+Lithium or Valproate (Berk et al. 2008) have been investigated in controlled studies and have positive evidence. Other combinations are either not studied under controlled conditions or have shown inconsistent results (Grunze et al., 2010).

4.3. Bipolar disorder prophylaxis

In routine practice, combination treatments are regularly employed to enhance efficacy of maintenance treatment and to address sub-syndromal symptoms or functional impairment.

http://dx.doi.org/10.5772/59004

Combination and Augmentation Treatments	Category of Evidence	Recommendation Grade
Olanzapine + Fluoxetine	Limited positive evidence from controlled studies	3
Lamotrigine + Lithium	Limited positive evidence from controlled studies	3
Modafinil + ongoing treatment	Limited positive evidence from controlled studies	3
N-acetylcysteine + Lithium or Valproate	Limited positive evidence from controlled studies	3
Sertraline + Lithium or Valproate	Evidence from uncontrolled studies	4
Tranylcypromine + ongoing treatment	Evidence from uncontrolled studies	4
Venlafaxine + Lithium or Valproate	Evidence from uncontrolled studies	4
L-Thyroxine + ongoing treatment	Evidence from uncontrolled studies	4
Topiramate + Lithium or Valproate	Evidence from uncontrolled studies	4
Zonisamide + Lithium or Valproate	Evidence from uncontrolled studies	4
Imipramine + Lithium	Inconsistent results	5
Inositol + Lithium or Valproate	Inconsistent results	5
Omega 3 fatty acids + Lithium or Valproate	Inconsistent results	5
Paroxetine + Lithium or Valproate	Inconsistent results	5
Bupropion + Lithium or Valproate	Inconsistent results	5
Gabapentin + ongoing treatment	Inconsistent results	5

Table 2. Categories of evidence and grades of recommendation for acute bipolar depression (Adapted from Grunze et al.(2010))

For example, prospective data of the Stanley Foundation Bipolar Network showed that over 55% of bipolar patients were on two or three medications, 31.8% required four or more drugs and 13.8% requiring five or more medications, but still it took a mean time of 1.5 years to achieve a sustained remission (Post et al., 2010). Positive placebo-controlled RCTs exist for combination treatments of mood stabilizers-valproate+lithium (Geddes et al., 2010), valproate or lithium, with all atypical antipsychotics that have a license for bipolar maintenance treatment – aripiprazole (Marcus et al., 2011), quetiapine (Vieta et al.,2008; Suppes et al., 2009), risperidone (Yatham et al., 2003) and ziprasidone (Bowden et al., 2010). The treatment of bipolar disorder patients may also change frequently in response to side effects, emerging comorbidities including physical health issues and other needs to be specifically tailored for each patient. These needs in real world patients are virtually impossible to capture in a guideline whose focus is the efficacy of a given combination treatment over a limited time period and in a fair proportion of patients. These limitations should be kept in mind when interpreting data of randomized controlled combination maintenance studies. For this reason, various guidelines do not make a special note or recommendation for specific combination treatments (Grunze et al., 2013).

5. Anxiety disorder

Benzodiazepines are used in combination with serotonergic drugs during the initial phase-a week or two, before the onset of anti-anxiety effect, either to hasten its efficacy or to suppress the activating side effects that are seen when serotonergic therapy has been started. In the treatment of panic disorder, there is persistent positive evidence from randomized controlled studies for the combination of antidepressants and benzodiazepines (clonazepam plus paroxetine or sertraline) (Pollack et al. 2003; Goddard et al. 2001). But evidence for other combinations is only from uncontrolled studies or case reports. Combination of antidepressants and benzodiazepines also has positive results from controlled data in the management of generalized anxiety disorder and social anxiety disorder. Combination of SSRI and atypical antipsychotics in the treatment of generalized anxiety disorder too has positive evidence from controlled trials (Bandelow et al., 2008). Although an array of combination, adjuvant, augmentation strategies are proposed for the treatment of OCD and PTSD, especially treatment resistance, only augmentation of SSRI with antipsychotics has positive evidence from controlled studies (Bandelow et al., 2008). Rest of the evidence is from uncontrolled data. Table 3 shows various combination regimens in the treatment of anxiety disorders with the recommendation grades.

Diagnosis	Combination and Augmentation Treatments	Category of Evidence	Recommendation Grade
PANIC DISORDER	1. Antidepressants + Benzodiazepines	Full evidence from controlled studies	2
	2. SSRIs+TCAs 3. SSRI+Olanzapine 4. SSRI+Pindolol or TCAs 5. Valproate+Clonazepam	Evidence from uncontrolled studies	4
	6. Lithium+Clomipramine	Evidence from case reports	4
GAD	1. Antidepressants+ Benzodiazepines	Full evidence from controlled studies	2
	2. SSRI+atypical antipsychotics (risperidone or olanzapine)	Limited positive evidence from controlled studies	3
SOCIAL PHOBIA	1. Antidepressants+ Benzodiazepines	Limited positive evidence from controlled studies	3
	2. SSRI+Buspirone	Evidence from uncontrolled studies	4
OCD	1. SSRI+antipsychotics(haloperidol, quetiapine, olanzapine and risperidone)	Limited positive evidence from controlled studies	3
	2. Citalopram+Reboxetine 3. SSRI+Clomipramine 4. Clomipramine+Lithium	Evidence from uncontrolled studies	4

http://dx.doi.org/10.5772/59004

Diagnosis	Combination and Augmentation Treatments	Category of Evidence	Recommendation Grade
	5. SSRI+Buspirone 6. SSRI+Topiramate 7. Clomipramine+L-tryptophan 8. SSRI+Pindolol+L-tryptophan		
PTSD	1. Adjunctive olanzapine or risperidone	Limited positive evidence from controlled studies	3
	2. SSRI+Triiodothyronine 3. Imipramine+Clonidine	Evidence from uncontrolled studies	4
	4. Venlafaxine+Quetiapine 5. SSRI+Gabapentin	Evidence from case reports	4

Table 3. Categories of evidence and grades of recommendation for anxiety disorders (Adapted from Bandelow et al. (2008))

6. Schizophrenia

Even on antipsychotic therapy patients with schizophrenia achieving full remission are only about 30% (Hert et al., 2007). Although clozapine has significantly greater efficacy compared to other antipsychotics when unresponsive to either typical or an atypical antipsychotic when used first, its use is associated with significant adverse effects (Kane et al., 1988). Combination therapy is one of the strategies to manage such unresponsiveness. Polypharmacy therapy in the treatment of schizophrenia might be either antipsychotics' combination or an antipsychotic combined with an agent not used primarily for treatment of psychosis but has an augmentative effect. It was observed that at baseline, many schizophrenia patients included in the Clinical Antipsychotic Trials of Intervention Effectiveness (CATIE) trial were on poly-pharmacotherapy-4% taking lithium, 15% other mood stabilizers, 38% antidepressants, 22% anxiolytics and 6% two antipsychotics (Chakos et al., 2006).

Mood stabilizers like lithium, carbamazepine and valproate have been used as adjuvants to antipsychotic treatment in schizophrenia. While randomized trial-based evidence is available for valproate and carbamazepine, no randomized controlled trials have investigated the effect of lithium in patients with schizophrenia. Patients receiving lithium augmentation showed clinically significant response; this significance was however lost when only patients with non affective symptoms were included (Leucht et al., 2007a). Data based on randomised trials suggests that there is no conclusive evidence to recommend either valproate or carbamazepine is useful as an adjunctive therapy in schizophrenia treatment. However in patients with schizophrenia, positive effects on aggression and tardive dyskinesia with valproate and on violence and EEG abnormalities with carbamazepine have been found (Leucht et al., 2007b; Schwarz et al., 2008).

None of the studies investigating the effect of other augmentation strategies like benzodiazepines, beta-blockers, antidepressants, anti-inflammatory agents, glutamatergic agents, and electroconvulsive therapy have been able to demonstrate significant improvement in patients with schizophrenia (Correll et al., 2009). Correll et al. (2009) identified certain clinical situations where antipsychotic co-treatment i.e. combining two antipsychotics are superior to antipsychotic monotherapy. Both acute exacerbations and chronically continuous course, co-starting second antipsychotic when compared to augmentation and, co-treatment including clozapine when compared to a strategy not including clozapine, have been found significant improvements in clinical symptomatology when managed with antipsychotic co-treatment than with monotherapy. Among the types of combinations: co-treatment with a typical agent and an atypical agent has been found to be better than a combination of either two typical or atypical agents. In a recent review, Ballon and Stroup (2013) question the generalizability of these findings by commenting that these significant effects would disappear with exclusion of studies from China. We agree to their remark on doubtfulness of replicating the in-vitro model that presumes modulating the schizophrenia pathophysiology at a receptor level citing the limitations in conducting proper clinical trials. Moreover, no guidelines suggest comparative evidence of individual molecules.

Moreover, evidence for efficacy of clozapine augmentation is also currently sparse. Efficacy of adjunctive AEDs like lamotrigine and topiramate, SSRIs like citalopram and co-treatment with other antipsychotics like sulpiride is based on single studies, that too with inconsistent findings (Sommer et al., 2012). Despite their popularity, pharmacological augmentations of clozapine are yet to be demonstrated to be superior to placebo. However, a recent metaanalysis, supports clozapine augmentation with amisulpride and aripiprazole, mirtazapine and ethyl eicosapentaenoic acid (Porcelli et al., 2012).

7. Substance use disorders

7.1. Alcohol use disorders

Antipsychotics, especially haloperidol, have been used in combination with a BZD for treatment of severe agitation in alcohol withdrawal delirium (Mayo-Smith et al. 2004); however there are no placebo-controlled trials available. Carbamazepine in combination with tiapride has also been found to be effective in treatment of this condition (Soyka et al., 2006). Although, minimal amount of evidence is available, antipsychotic treatment in combination with benzodiazepines is warranted in the treatment of alcohol related psychosis (Soyka et al., 2011). For relapse prevention, disulfiram is considered a second-line medication that can be combined with either naltrexone or acamprosate (Soyka et al., 2011). Although positive open trials are present (Feeney et al. 2006), a recent controlled trial, COMBINE failed to show that acamprosate is effective in relapse prevention, either alone, or in combination with naltrexone (Anton et al. 2006). Ait-Daoudet al. (2001) found combination of ondansetron and naltrexone reduces craving.

http://dx.doi.org/10.5772/59004

7.2. Opioid use disorders

A combination of naloxone and flumazenil has been shown to be significantly effective in treating opioid intoxication with additional benzodiazepine use (Megarbane et al., 2010). Commonly used combination of clonidine and naltrexone has been regarded as safe and effective for rapid detoxification (Kleber et al. 2007). More importantly, combination of buprenorphine and naloxone has excellent evidence in the treatment of opioid withdrawal. Evidence also supports the use of clonidine and lofexidine as adjunctive medications (Soyka et al., 2011).

8. Epilepsy

Initial treatment of epilepsies is usually a single antiepileptic drug. However in resistant cases, strategies like alternate monotherapy or polytherapy are suggested. As alternative monotherapy is less common because of the limited efficacy and possible side effects of drugs, polytherapy is commonly initiated when monotherapy fails to control seizures (Bauer et al., 1998). Although there is satisfactory evidence on initial monotherapy, data on long term effectiveness or subsequent polypharmacy regimens is lacking; more so with older antiepileptic drugs (AEDs). Trials have shown that adjunctive therapy with newer AEDs (levetiracetam, oxcarbazepine and topiramate) was favorable than when compared to placebo (Wilby et al., 2005). Costa et al (2011) in a systematic review and meta-analysis of trials comparing a new add-on antiepileptic drug treatment with placebo or drug, found a relatively small magnitude to allow a definitive conclusion about which new antiepileptic drug has superior effectiveness. However these trials are of short duration and often fail to limit inclusion to either partial or generalised seizures. Adjunctive treatment with benzodiazepines also has a poor fund of evidence.

9. Child and geriatric populations

One third of pharmacologically treated mentally ill children and adolescents receive polypharmacy, with a remarkable increase in the number of children receiving two or more medications in the past decade (McIntyre and Jerell, 2009)

Psychiatric polypharmacy is common in child and adolescent and geriatric population as well. With a prevalence of multi-class polypharmacy in child and adolescent population to be 19%, antidepressants are the most commonly co-prescribed drugs followed by attention deficit and hyperactivity disorder (ADHD) medications, antipsychotics, mood stabilizers and benzodiazepines (Comer et al., 2010). Except for a few open label studies (Kowatch et al., 2003), data from randomized controlled trials is lacking in this group. Interactions between the various molecules in childhood disorders are remarkable. While methylphenidate did not improve symptoms of ADHD compared to placebo in children and adolescents with bipolar disorder stabilized on aripiprazole, this agent could improve ADHD symptoms in those taking lithium and valproate (Zigman and Blier, 2012). Such noteworthy interactions suggest empirical rational polypharmacy rather than evidence based polypharmacy.

Similar comment on geriatric population also can be made. Psychiatric polypharmacy in this population is very common (Loyola et al., 2008) and the major reason for such an approach is the presence of medical comorbidities, where evidence base is intricate to build.

9.1. Dementia

Polypharmacy in the treatment of dementia has some evidence base. The rational is that combination therapy of drugs with different modes of action might have a synergistic effect (Ihl et al., 2011). There are randomized controlled trials that investigated the efficacy of combination of memantine with various cholinesterase inhibitors and galantamine. However, there is no conclusive evidence as these studies report both positive and negative results (Dantoine et al., 2006, Ihl et al., 2011, Kornhuber et al., 2009, Porsteinsson et al., 2008). There is some evidence from uncontrolled open studies on the effect of donepezil and gingko biloba combination, but negative (Yancheva et al., 2007).

10. Medical comorbidity

Polypharmacy in patients with medical comorbidity is a rule, however, evidence based pharmacological treatment in such conditions is very scarce, in fact less applicable. One important reason is that these subjects are not eligible for most clinical trials (Zimmerman et al., 2002). It is difficult to conduct randomized controlled trials on these subjects as there would be obvious complicatedness in setting the inclusion and exclusion criteria. It is recommended that clinicians should opt for individualized or empirical polypharmacy.

11. Individualized rational polypharmacy

Kingsbury et al. (2001) divided rational polypharmacy into two types: validated and empirical. Validation or evidence base is based on results from controlled trials or meta-analyses. These results guide treatment presuming homogeneity in the illnesses, which hardly exists. Empirical rational polypharmacy is more individualized. Hence empirically this classification can be restated into "standardized" and "individualized" rational polypharmacy. Standardized rational polypharmacy refers to the validated strategies that have been discussed so far. Individualized rational polypharmacy is based on a complete evaluation of the index patient-timing and characterization of various manifestations, a proper evaluation of response to drugs in other affected family members and conducting mini investigations in the background of adequate knowledge of pharmacogenomics, receptor profiles and rating of psychopathology. Clinicians with proper training and motivation only could go ahead with this strategy; otherwise these tactics would end up in contra-therapeutic polypharmacy.

http://dx.doi.org/10.5772/59004

12. Causes of irrational polypharmacy and ways to tackle them

Apart from practicing rational polypharmacy, clinicians need to understand various reasons and ways to tackle irrational polypharmacy. Several different causes of irrational polypharmacy have been identified (Kingsbury et al., 2001):

1. Fear and laziness. Continuing the earlier prescribed drug/s that has/have not shown improvement along with the later drug after addition of which there is some response; continuing the drug that was added to ameliorate acute symptoms even after the primary drug's later onset of action has begun.

2. Sloppy diagnosis/ overdiagnosis: such as that of schizoaffective for affective symptoms which could be a part of schizophrenia or for psychotic agitation misdiagnosing it as an affective manifestation.

3. Improper titration. Mistaking the effect of the second drug to be due to a combination of both amidst of the cross titration process.

4. Blind adherence to maximum doses. 80% response on 'x' dose of a dose (that is considered maximum according to one particular guideline) is added with another drug (even after knowing '2x' dose of the first drug could have been tolerated).

5. Inadequate awareness/ blind disbelief on the therapeutic efficacy of psychotherapeutic strategies

6. Inadequate knowledge or inattention towards receptor profile of the molecules.

7. Adhering to industry sponsored guidelines

8. Magical beliefs/ using methods based on word of mouth.

Apart from these causes, industry driven pressure leading to unethical practice and improper monitoring of drug compliance are also equally responsible for irrational polypharmacy. Zigman and Blier (2012) consider pharmacological characteristics like redundancy (two or more drugs have similar/overlapping mechanism of action), pharmacodynamic and pharmacokinetic interactions also as causes of irrational polypharmacy. Zigman and Blier (2012) also provide certain strategies to tackle irrational polypharmacy.

Firstly, to consider selectively active or multifunctional medications wherever appropriate. Two medications selectively active at two different receptors can be chosen when their action at these receptors is known to improve the clinical condition, whereas two multifunctional medications having more or less similar profile at the target receptor should be avoided in combination. Secondly, to consider various pharmacodynamic and pharmacokinetic interactions of the molecules in use. An acetylcholinesterase inhibitor should be avoided in combination with a drug with potent anticholinergic side effects, whereas using a drug in combination with a cytochrome p450 enzyme inducer reduces the efficacy of the drug and lead to irrational polypharmacy. Another strategy is to allow for adequate dose and duration before considering adjunctive or augmentative strategies. Such strategies although scientific, when used without the adequate trial of a previous drug, would be labeled irrational. The last strategy is to regularly reassess the efficacy of the ongoing combination treatment. Moreover, a trial of tapering one of the drugs in the combination should be given when the response is adequate and has sustained for a period of time.

Niculescu and Hulvershorn (2010) suggest a personalized tri-dimensional treatment (i.e., concurrent treatment of anxiety, mood, and cognitive abnormalities) plus modulation of environmental factors (e.g., stress). Such an approach involves rational polypharmacy—the combination of three or more medications, each acting primarily on anxiety, mood, or cognition, respectively. Depending on the major pathology, one of these medications is used at a higher dose and the others at lower doses. For example, in schizophrenia, an antipsychotic may be primary at a higher dose, with an anxiolytic and/or mood stabilizer secondary at lower doses. Similarly for mood abnormalities such as bipolar disorder, a mood stabilizer at a higher dose would be the primary approach and an anxiolytic and antipsychotic secondary at lower doses.

Apart from these measures, thorough evaluation of the patient's clinical symptoms and medication history along with assessment of drug compliance is of utmost importance in managing irrational polypharmacy. Obtaining drug levels where applicable and a thorough evaluation of reasons for treatment resistance including ruling out general medical causes is another important action to avoid irrational polypharmacy and provide maximum patient care.

Although not validated, polypharmacy justification checklist, not only to justify rational polypharmacy but also to curb irrational polypharmacy, has been generated by Dr. Clif Tennison, Helen Ross McNabb Center, East Tennessee. It is a 38 item checklist targeting 9 domains (Appendix).

13. Indian context

There is some epidemiological data available on psychiatric polypharmacy from India. Polypharmacy is common in India and its prevalence rates range from 9-73% (Padmini et al., 2007; Sawhney et al., 2004). Ramadas et al. (2010) found that antipsychotic polypharmacy is more related to typical than with atypical agents. However recently, Shrivastava et al. (2012) found almost 30% of first episode schizophrenia patients receiving more than one atypical antipsychotic. These studies were limited to a section of geographical area and it would be difficult to generalize these findings to other parts of India. Indian studies that have compared the efficacy of rational polypharmacy with mono-therapies are however lacking. However, the Indian psychiatric society has formulated certain guidelines for combination therapies in various disorders. Although no direct recommendation is available, various comments are made on these regimens (Table 4).

http://dx.doi.org/10.5772/59004

Year	Disorder	Available evidence for polypharmacy regimens and comments
2005	Schizophrenia	• Combination of intramuscular haloperidol and lorazepam faster response than haloperidol alone • Adjunct studies in India – all open • Adjunctive medications recommended- Lithium carbonate; Antidepressants; Benzodiazepines; and Anticonvulsants. • No specific guidelines
2005	Depression	• Major depressive disorder with psychotic features require combined use of antidepressant and antipsychotic medication especially fluoxetine and olanzapine combination • An SSRI combined with a TCA induce rapid antidepressant response • First strategy for resistant depression- augmentation with Lithium/Thyroid/Buspirone; next: combination (TCA-SSRI. Bupropion-SSRI) Depression with anxiety: Efficacy of high potency benzodiazepine like alprazolam and clonazepam in combination with antidepressants is beneficial
2005	Bipolar disorder	• Valproate plus haloperidol superior antipsychotic alone in reduction of manic symptoms • Difficulty in assessing benzodiazepine combination due to short treatment durations, distinguishing specific antimanic effects from nonspecific sedative effects. • Lithium plus an antipsychotic and valproate plus an antipsychotic suggest greater efficacy or a more rapid onset of action than with these agents alone • Combination of divalproex plus an SSRI an effective strategy for management of breakthrough depression during maintenance of bipolar I disorder
2006	Alcohol use disorders	• Several animal studies demonstrate combinations of medications e.g. disulfiram +naltraxone, acamprosate +naltraxone are more effective in reducing alcohol intake than these drugs used alone • Myth: Combining more than one treatment method has no advantage.
2006	Nicotine use dirorders	• Combining nicotine patch with either nicotine gum or nicotine nasal spray increases long-term abstinence rates over those produced by a single form of nicotine replacement therapy
2006	Opioid use disorders	• In the management of withdrawal, non opioid medications like clonidine, benzodiazepines, NSAIDs or a combination of these. • Rapid detoxification: Naloxone in combination with other medications such as clonidine and benzodiazepines • Naltrexone with clonidine for rapid detoxification is safe and effective • Buprenorphine and naloxone combination utilized for agonist maintenance therapy
2007	Elderly anxiety disorders	• Benzodiazepines may be used to reduce the severity of anxiety, the need for rapid anxiolysis along with SSRIs • Beta blockers may be used as augmenting agents, especially when somatic symptoms of anxiety are prominent • Low dose of a tricyclic antidepressant could be used to treat insomnia associated with anxiety in patients who are receiving SSRI.
2007	Alzheimer's disease	• The use and combinations of pharmacological agents should be decided on a case-by-case basis.

Year	Disorder	Available evidence for polypharmacy regimens and comments
2007	Elderly depression	• Patients with major depression with psychotic features require combined use of antidepressant and antipsychotic medications
2007	Psychosis in elderly	• Refractory cases may be tried on a combination of clozapine + Amisulpride. • Lithium augmentation, citalopram+methylphenidate, modafinil+floxetine or mirtazapine, dexamethasone plus any antidepressant may be indicated
2008	Depression in children and Adolescents	• Recommendation for adults with TRD may be applicable to youth
2008	ADHD	• Combined pharmacotherapy only to be used when at least two individual agents (initially methylphenidate and dexamphetamine) have failed.

Table 4. Data on polypharmacy regimens in the Indian Psychiatric society treatment guidelines

14. Summary, conclusions and recommendations

- Following the dimensional approach in treating psychiatric disorders, polypharmacy, specifically, multiclass polypharmacy is very common.
- However, rationality in the approach determines whether the outcome is therapeutic or contra therapeutic.
- A positive evidence base from controlled trials for polypharmacy is highest for-
- Depression (add on)-mirtazapine in combination with SSRI
- Depression (augment)-SSRI s with atypical antipsychotics/lithium
- Acute mania-there is not enough unambiguous evidence that supports combination therapy of antipsychotic+mood stabilizer as a general first line treatment.
- Acute bipolar depression-olanzapine+fluoxetine and lamotrigine+lithium
- Bipolar prophylaxis-valproate+lithium, valproate or lithium, with atypical antipsychotics (aripiprazole, quetiapine, risperidone and ziprasidone).
- Panic disorder-combination of clonazepam plus paroxetine or sertraline.
- Generalized anxiety disorder-combination of antidepressants and benzodiazepines and combination of SSRI and atypical antipsychotics
- Social anxiety disorder-combination of antidepressants and benzodiazepines
- OCD & PTSD-augmentation of SSRI with antipsychotics
- Schizophrenia-valproate and carbamazepine adjuvant treatment; clozapine augmentation with amisulpride and aripiprazole, mirtazapine and ethyl eicosapentaenoic acid
- Alcohol withdrawal delirium-haloperidol used in combination with a BZD

http://dx.doi.org/10.5772/59004

- Opioid withdrawal-naloxone and flumazenil, buprenorphine and naloxone; rapid detoxification-clonidine and naltrexone;
- Focal epilepsies-adjunctive therapy with newer AEDs (levetiracetam, oxcarbazepine and topiramate)
- It is recommended that clinicians should opt for individualized or empirical polypharmacy as it is difficult to conduct randomized controlled trials on these subjects because of obvious complicatedness in setting the inclusion and exclusion criteria and derive/ generalize data from them.
- Use of polypharmacy justification checklist to justify rational polypharmacy and also to curb irrational polypharmacy may be an useful option

Abbreviations

- 5HT1A-5-hydroxytryptamine 1A
- ADHD-Attention Deficit and Hyperactivity Disorder
- AED-Anti Epileptic Drug
- BZD-Benzodiazepine
- CATIE-Clinical Antipsychotic Trials of Intervention Effectiveness
- EEG-Electroencephalography
- GSK-Glycogen synthase kinase
- MAO-Monoamine oxidase
- NIMH-National Institute of Mental Health
- NSAID-Non-steroidal anti-inflammatory drug
- OCD-Obsessive Compulsive Disorder
- PTSD-Post Traumatic Stress Disorder
- RCT-Randomized Control Trial
- SAM-S-adenosyl-l-methionine
- SNRI-Serotonin–norepinephrine reuptake inhibitor
- SSRI-selective serotonin reuptake inhibitor
- TCA-Tricyclic Antidepressant
- TRD-Treatment Resistant Depression
- U.S. FDA-The United States Food and Drug Administration

Appendix

POLYPHARMACY JUSTIFICATION CHECKLIST

	YES	NO
1. Before prescribing polypharmacy:		
a. Thorough evaluation of clinical presentation?	☐	☐
b. Thorough evaluation of diagnosis?	☐	☐
2. Evaluation of medication history:		
a. Efficacy of past medications documented/reviewed?	☐	☐
b. Reported side effects of past medications documented/reviewed?	☐	☐
c. Dose and duration of past monotherapy attempts documented/reviewed?	☐	☐
i. At least 21 days of continuous use at same dose? (Mood stabilizers and antipsychotics may require longer trials.)	☐	☐
ii. 2-to-3 monotherapy trials with drugs from different classes?	☐	☐
iii. Review of diagnosis after failure of several monotherapy trials?	☐	☐
3. Patient compliance:		
a. Review of patient compliance during medication trial(s) documented?	☐	☐
b. Patient involvement in reviewing treatment response and treatment options?	☐	☐
c. Review of simplicity of regimen and avoiding complicated regimen?	☐	☐
4. Evaluation of the current medication regimen:		
a. Rationale for each current medication reviewed?	☐	☐
b. Efficacy of each current medication reviewed?	☐	☐
c. OTC medications, herbal remedies, and illicit drugs reviewed?	☐	☐
d. One-time orders and prn medications reviewed? (If >3/week for 3-4 weeks, these should be considered part of a patient's scheduled medication regimen).	☐	☐
5. Review of medication changes:		
a. Total number of medications reduced before adding new one?	☐	☐
b. Only one medication changed at a time?	☐	☐
c. Medication changes completed? Old medication discontinued after new one at therapeutic level for sufficient period of time?	☐	☐
d. Cross-titrations used only with those medications for which this strategy is required?	☐	☐
6. Demonstrable need:		
a. Medications without clear benefit for target symptoms eliminated?	☐	☐
7. Combined and Augmented Pharmacotherapy:		
a. Justification for same-class polypharmacy clearly documented?	☐	☐
i. Specific targeting of different symptom clusters?	☐	☐
ii. Synergism in the drugs' mechanisms of action?	☐	☐
iii. Augmentation of partial treatment response or nonresponse to monotherapy?	☐	☐
iv. Improved risk/benefit ratio by reducing dosage and adverse effects for improved tolerability of one or both drugs?	☐	☐
b. Failed trials of monotherapy documented?	☐	☐
c. Efficacy data on strategically combined treatments reviewed?	☐	☐
8. Monitoring the risks of polypharmacy:		
a. Drug interactions reviewed?	☐	☐
b. Blood levels monitored periodically, especially with signs of toxicity or with medications likely to have drug interactions?	☐	☐
c. Monitoring of higher-risk combinations:		
i. More than one medication from the same class?	☐	☐
ii. More than two antipsychotic medications?	☐	☐
iii. Combinations with cumulative anticholinergic effects?	☐	☐
iv. Combinations with specific additive organ or system effects? (e.g., Cardiac, Renal, Hepatic, Respiratory, Gastrointestinal, Musculoskeletal)	☐	☐
9. Institutional mechanisms in place:		
a. Peer review	☐	☐
b. Automatic/forced drug interaction reviews	☐	☐
c. Supported access to medication information	☐	☐
d. Pharmacy consultation	☐	☐
e. Drug utilization review	☐	☐

http://dx.doi.org/10.5772/59004

Author details

S. Haque Nizamie* and Sai Krishna Tikka

*Address all correspondence to: sh.nizamie@gmail.com

Central Institute of Psychiatry, Ranchi, India

References

[1] Ait-Daoud N, Johnson BA, Prohoda TJ, Hargita ID. 2001. Combining ondansetron and naltrexone reduces craving among biologically predisposed alcoholics: preliminary clinical evidence. Psychopharmacology 154:2327.

[2] Alpert JE, Papakostas G, Mischoulon D, et al. S-Adenosyl-Lmethionine (SAMe) as an adjunct for resistant major depressive disorder: an open trial following partial or nonresponse to selective serotonin reuptake inhibitors or venlafaxine. J Clin Psychopharmacol 2004;24:661–4.

[3] Andrade C, Kharawala S. Practice guideline for the pharmacological treatment of anxiety disorders in the elderly. Indian psychiatric society treatment guidelines 2007.

[4] Anton RF, O'Malley SS, Ciraulo DA, et al. 2006. Combined pharmacotherapies and behavioural interventions for alcohol dependence: the Combine study: a randomized controlled trial. J Am Med Assoc 295:20032017.

[5] Avasthi A, Grover S, Bharadwaj R. Clinical Practice Guidelines for Treatment of Depression in Elderly. Indian psychiatric society treatment guidelines 2007.

[6] Avasthi A, Kumar S, Vikas A. Clinical practice guidelines for the management of bipolar affective (mood) disorders. Indian psychiatric society treatment guidelines 2005.

[7] Awasti A. Treatment of Depression in Children and Adoescents. Indian psychiatric society treatment guidelines 2008.

[8] Ballon J, Stroup TS. Polypharmacy for schizophrenia. Curr Opin Psychiatry 2013;26(2):208-13.

[9] Bandelow B, Zohar J, Hollander E, Kasper S, Möller HJ. World Federation of Societies of Biological Psychiatry (WFSBP) guidelines for the pharmacological treatment of anxiety, obsessive-compulsive and post-traumatic stress disorders-first revision.World J Biol Psychiatry. 2008;9(4):248-312.

[10] Baruch P, Filteau MJ, Bouchard RH, Pourcher E, Vincent P, Jouvent R. The dimensional approach to clinical psychopharmacology: a polysemous concept. J Psychiatry Neurosci. 1992;17(2):55-60.

[11] Basan A, Kissling W, Leucht S. Valproate as an adjunct to antipsychotics for schizophrenia: a systematic review of randomized trials. Schizophr Res. 2004;70(1):33–37.

[12] Bauer J. Anticonvulsant combination therapy: rational concepts versus real effectiveness. Fortschr Neurol Psychiatr 1998;66:414-426.

[13] Bauer M, Adli M, Bschor T (2010) Lithium's emerging role in the treatment of refractory major depressive episodes: augmentation of antidepressants. Neuropsychobiology 62: 36–42.

[14] Berk M, Copolov DL, Dean O, Lu K, Jeavons S, Schapkaitz I,et al. 2008. N-Acetyl cysteine for depressive symptoms in bipolardisorder– a double-blind randomized placebo-controlledtrial. Biol Psychiatry 64:468–475.

[15] Blier P, Gobbi G, Turcotte JE, de Montigny C, Boucher N, Hébert C, Debonnel G. Mirtazapine and paroxetine in major depression: a comparison of monotherapy versus their combination from treatment initiation. Eur Neuropsychopharmacol 2009; 19:457–465.

[16] Blier P, Ward HE, Tremblay P, Laberge L, Hébert C, Bergeron R. Combination of antidepressant medications from treatment initiation for major depressive disorder: a double-blind randomized study. Am J Psychiatry 2010; 167:281–288.

[17] Bowden CL, Vieta E, Ice KS, Schwartz JH, Wang PP, Versavel M. Ziprasidone plus a mood stabilizer in subjects with bipolar I disorder: a 6-month, randomized, placebo-controlled, double-blind trial. J Clin Psychiatry 2010;71:130–7.

[18] Brown E, Dunner DL, McElroy SL, Keck PE, Adams DH,Degenhardt E, et al. 2009. Olanzapine/fluoxetine combinationvs. lamotrigine in the 6-month treatment of bipolar I depression.Int J Neuropsychopharmacol 12(6):773–782.

[19] Carpenter LL, Yasmin S, Price LH. A double-blind, placebo-controlled study of antidepressant augmentation with mirtazapine. Biol Psychiatry 2002; 51:183–188.

[20] Chakos MH, Glick ID, Miller AL, Hamner MB, Miller DD, Patel JK, et al. Baseline use of concomitant psychotropic medications to treat schizophrenia in the CATIE trial. Psychiatr Serv. 2006;57:1094–101.

[21] Comer JS, Olfson M, Mojtabai R. National trends in child and adolescent psychotropic polypharmacy in office-based practice, 1996-2007. J Am Acad Child Adolesc Psychiatry 2010;49:1001–10.

[22] Connolly KR, Thase ME. If at first you don't succeed: a review of the evidence for antidepressant augmentation, combination and switching strategies. Drugs 2011;71(1):43-64.

[23] Correll CU, Rummel-Kluge C, Corves C, Kane JM, Leucht S. Antipsychotic combinations vs monotherapy in schizophrenia: a meta-analysis of randomized controlled trials. Schizophr Bull 2009;35(2):443-57.

[24] Costa J, Fareleira F, Ascenção R, Borges M, Sampaio C, Vaz-Carneiro A. Clinical comparability of the new antiepileptic drugs in refractory partial epilepsy: a systematic review and meta-analysis. Epilepsia 2011;52:1280-91.

[25] Dantoine T, Auriacombe S, Sarazin M, Becker H, Pere JJ, Bourdeix I. 2006. Rivastigmine monotherapy and combination therapy with memantine in patients with moderately severe Alzheimer'sdisease who failed to benefi t from previous cholinesterase inhibitor treatment. Int J Clin Pract 60:110 – 118.

[26] De las Cuevas C, Sanz EJ. Polypharmacy in psychiatric practice in the Canary Islands. BMC Psychiatry 2004;4:18.

[27] Desai NG, Kumar R, Sengupta SN, Sharma P. Clinical practice guidelines for treatment of alcohol dependence. Indian psychiatric society treatment guidelines 2006.

[28] Feeney GFX, Connor JP, Young McD, Tucker J, McPherson A. 2006. Combined acamprosate and naltrexone, with cognitive behavioral therapy is superior to either medication alone for alcohol abstinence: A single centre's experience with pharmacotherapy. Alcohol Alcoholism 41:321327.

[29] Findling RL, Short EJ, McNamara NK, et al. (2007) Methylphenidate in the treatment of children and adolescents with bipolar disorder and attention-deficit/hyperactivity disorder. J Am Acad Child Adolesc Psychiatry 46: 1445–1453.

[30] Frye MA, Grunze H, Suppes T, McElroy SL, Keck PE, Walden J,et al. 2007. A placebo-controlled evaluation of adjunctivemodafi nil in the treatment of bipolar depression.Am J Psychiatry164:1242–1249.

[31] Frye MA, Ketter TA, Leverich GS, Huggins T, Lantz C, Denicoff KD, Post R. The increasing use of polypharmacotherapy for refractory mood disorders: 22 years of study. J Clin Psychiatry 2000;61:9–15.

[32] Gautam S, Batra L, Gaur N, Meena PS. Clinical Practice Guidelines for the Assessment and Treatment of Attention-Deficit/Hyperactivity Disorder. Indian psychiatric society treatment guidelines. Indian psychiatric society treatment guidelines 2008.

[33] Gautam S, Batra L, Gawri A. Clinical practice guidelines for management of nicotine dependence. Indian psychiatric society treatment guidelines 2006.

[34] Gautam S, Batra L. Clinical practice guidelines for the management of depression. Indian psychiatric society treatment guidelines 2005.

[35] Gautam S, Bhatia G, Khan A, Odha PI, Gaur N. Clinical practice guidelines on psychoses in elderly. Indian psychiatric society treatment guidelines 2007.

[36] Gautam S, Gupta ID, Nijhawan A, Gaur V. Clinical practice guidelines for management of opioid dependence. Indian psychiatric society treatment guidelines 2006.

[37] Geddes JR, Goodwin GM, Rendell J, et al. (2010) Lithium plus valproate combination therapy versus monotherapy for relapse prevention in bipolar I disorder (BALANCE): a randomised open-label trial. Lancet 375: 385–395.

[38] Glauser T, Ben-Menachem E, Bourgeois B, Cnaan A, Guerreiro C, Kälviäinen R, Mattson R, French JA, Perucca E, Tomson T. Updated ILAE evidence review of antiepileptic drug efficacy and effectiveness as initial monotherapy for epileptic seizures and syndromes. Epilepsia 2013;54:551-563.

[39] Goddard AW, Brouette T, Almai A, Jetty P, Woods SW, CharneyD. 2001. Early coadministration of clonazepam with sertralinefor panic disorder. Arch Gen Psychiatry 58:681686.

[40] Grunze H, Vieta E, Goodwin GM, Bowden C, Licht RW, Moller HJ, Kasper S.The World Federation of Societies of Biological Psychiatry (WFSBP) guidelines for the biological treatment of bipolar disorders: update 2009 on the treatment of acute mania.World J Biol Psychiatry 2009;10(2):85-116.

[41] Grunze H, Vieta E, Goodwin GM, Bowden C, Licht RW, Möller HJ, Kasper S. The World Federation of Societies of Biological Psychiatry (WFSBP) Guidelines for the Biological Treatment of Bipolar Disorders: Update 2010 on the treatment of acute bipolar depression.World J Biol Psychiatry 2010;11(2):81-109.

[42] Grunze H, Vieta E, Goodwin GM, Bowden C, Licht RW, Möller HJ, Kasper S. The World Federation of Societies of Biological Psychiatry (WFSBP) guidelines for the biological treatment of bipolar disorders: update 2012 on the long-term treatment of bipolar disorder.World J Biol Psychiatry 2013;14(3):154-219.

[43] Hert MD, van Winkel R, Wampers M, et al. Remission criteria for schizophrenia: evaluation in a large naturalistic cohort. Schizophr Res 2007; 92:68–73.

[44] Ihl R, Frölich L, Winblad B, Schneider L, Burns A, Möller HJ. World Federation of Societies of Biological Psychiatry (WFSBP) guidelines for the biological treatment of Alzheimer's disease and other dementias. World J Biol Psychiatry. 2011 Feb;12(1): 2-32.

[45] Kane JM, Honigfeld G, Singer J, Meltzer H. Clozapine in treatment-resistant schizophrenics. Psychopharmacol Bull. 1988; 24(1):62–67.

[46] Kingsbury SJ, Lotito ML. Psychiatric polypharmacy: the good, the bad, and the ugly. Psychiatric Times 2007;24(4):NP.

[47] Kingsbury SJ, Yi D, Simpson GM. Psychopharmacology: rational and irrational polypharmacy. Psychiatr Serv. 2001;52(8):1033-6.

[48] Kleber HD, Weiss RD, Anton RF Jr, George TP, Greenfi eld SF, Kosten TR, et al. 2007. Treatment of patients with substance use disorders, second edition. Am J Psychiatry 164:5 – 123.

[49] Kornhuber J, Schmidtke K, Frolich L, Perneczky R, Wolf S, Hampel H, et al. 2009. Early and differential diagnosis of dementia and mild cognitive impairment: design and cohort baseline characteristics of the German Dementia Competence Network. Dement Geriatr Cogn Disord 27:404 – 417 (Epub 1 April 2009).

[50] Kowatch RA, Sethuraman G, Hume JH, Kromelis M, Weinberg WA. Combination Pharmacotherapy in Children and Adolescents with Bipolar Disorder. Biol Psychiatry 2003;53:978–984.

[51] Kukreja S, Kalra G, Shah N, Shrivastava A. Polypharmacy in psychiatry: a review. Mens Sana Monogr. 2013;11(1):82-99.

[52] Kulhara P, Chakrabarti S. Clinical practice guidelines for the management of schizophrenia. Indian psychiatric society treatment guidelines 2005.

[53] Leucht S, Kissling W, McGrath J, White P. Carbamazepine for schizophrenia. Cochrane Database Syst Rev 2007b; Issue 3: CD001258.

[54] Leucht S, Kissling W, McGrath J. Lithium for schizophrenia. Cochrane Database Syst Rev 2007a; Issue 3: CD003834.

[55] Leucht S, McGrath J, Kissling W. Lithium for Schizophrenia (Cochrane Review). The Cochrane Library. 2003;Issue 3.

[56] Leucht S, McGrath J, White P, Kissling W. Carbamazapine for Schizophrenia and Schizoaffective Psychoses (Cochrane Review). The Cochrane Library. Issue 2.

[57] Liu P, He FF, Bai WP, et al. 2004. Menopausal depression: comparison of hormone replacement therapy and hormone replacement therapy plus fluoxetine. Chin Med J, 117:189–94.

[58] Loyola Filho AI, Uchoa E, Firmo JO, Lima-Costa MF. Influence of income on the association between cognitive impairment and polypharmacy: Bambuí Project. Rev Saude Publica 2008;42:89–99.

[59] Marcus R, Khan A, Rollin L, Morris B, Timko K, Carson W, Sanchez R. Efficacy of aripiprazole adjunctive to lithium or valproate in the long-term treatment of patients with bipolar I disorder with an inadequate response to lithium or valproate monotherapy: a multicenter, double-blind, randomized study. Bipolar Disord 2011;13:133–44.

[60] Mayo-Smith MF, Breecher LH, Fischer TL, et al. 2004. Management of alcohol withdrawal delirium. An evidence-based practice guideline. Arch Intern Med 164:14051412.

[61] McEvoy JP, Lieberman JA, Stroup TS, et al. Effectiveness of clozapine versus olanzapine, quetiapine, and risperidone in patients with chronic schizophrenia who did not respond to prior atypical antipsychotic treatment. Am J Psychiatry 2006;163:600–610.

[62] McIntyre RS, Jerrell JM. Polypharmacy in children and adolescents treated for major depressive disorder: a claims database study. J Clin Psychiatry 2009;70:240–246.

[63] Megarbane B, Buisien A, Jacobs F, Resiere D, Chevillard L, Vicaut E, Baud FJ. 2010. Prospective comparative assessment of buprenorphine overdose with heroin and methadone: clinical characteristics and response to antidotal treatment. J Subst Abuse Treat 38:403 – 407.

[64] Mojtabai R, Olfson M. National trends in psychotropic medication polypharmacy in office-based psychiatry. Arch Gen Psychiatry. 2010;67(1):26-36.

[65] Moret C. Combination/augmentation strategies for improving the treatment of depression. Neuropsychiatric disease and treatment 2005:1(4) 301–9.

[66] National Association of State Mental Health Program Directors (NASMHPD): Technical Report on Psychiatric Polypharmacy. Medical Directors Council and State Medicaid Directors: Alexandria, Virginia: 2001.

[67] Nelson JC and Papakostas GI. Atypical antipsychotic augmentation in major depressive disorder: a meta-analysis of placebo-controlled randomized trials. Am J Psychiatry 2009;166:980–91.

[68] Nelson JC, Mazure CM, Jatlow PI, et al. Combining norepinephrine and serotonin reuptake inhibition mechanisms for treatment of depression: a double-blind, randomized study. Biol Psychiatry 2004;55: 296–300.

[69] Niculescu AB, Hulvershorn LA. Toward Early, Personalized, Rational Polypharmacy In Psychiatry: A Tri-Dimensional Approach. Psychopharm Rev 2010; 45: 9-16.

[70] Padmini DD, Amarjeeth R, Sushma M, Guido S. Prescription patterns of psychotropic drugs in hospitalized schizophrenic patients in a tertiary care hospital. Calicut Med J. 2007;5:e3.

[71] Peh AL, Tay LK.Demographical profile and clinical features of patients with bipolar disorder in an outpatient setting in Singapore.Singapore Medical J 2008 May;49(5): 380-3.

[72] Perlis RH, Ostacher MJ, Patel JK, et al. Predictors of recurrence in bipolar disorder: primary outcomes from the Systematic Treatment Enhancement Program for Bipolar Disorder (STEP-BD). Am J Psychiatry 2006;163:217–224.

[73] Pollack MH, Simon NM, Worthington JJ, Doyle AL, Peters P,Toshkov F, et al. 2003b. Combined paroxetine and clonazepamtreatment strategies compared to paroxetine monotherapy forpanic disorder. J Psychopharmacol 17:276282.

[74] Porcelli S, Balzarro B, Serretti A. Clozapine resistance: augmentation strategies. Eur Neuropsychopharmacol 2012;22:165-182.

[75] Porsteinsson AP, Grossberg GT, Mintzer J, Olin JT, Memantine MEM-MD-12 Study Group. 2008. Memantine treatment in patients with mild to moderate Alzheimer's disease already receiving a cholinesterase inhibitor: a randomized, double-blind, placebo-controlled trial. Curr Alzheimer Res 5:83 – 89.

[76] Post RM, Altshuler LL, Frye MA, Suppes T, Keck PE Jr, McElroy SL, Leverich GS, Luckenbaugh DA, Rowe M, Pizzarello S, Kupka RW, Grunze H, Nolen WA.Complexity of pharmacologic treatment required for sustained improvement in outpatients with bipolar disorder.J Clin Psychiatry 2010;71(9):1176-86.

[77] Ramadas S, Kuttichira P, Sumesh TP, Ummer SA. A study of an antipsychotic prescription pattern of patients with schizophrenia in a developing country. Indian J Psychol Med 2010;32:13–6.

[78] Rush AJ, Trivedi MH, Wisniewski SR, et al. Acute and longer term outcomes in depressed outpatients requiring one or several treatment steps: a STAR*D report. Am J Psychiatry 2006;163:1905–1917.

[79] Rush AJ. Combining Antidepressant Medications: A Good Idea? Am J Psychiatry 2010;167:241-3.

[80] Sawhney V, Chopra V, Kapoor B, Thappa JR, Tandon VR. Prescription trends in schizophrenia and manic depressive psychosis. J K Sci. 2005;7:156–8.

[81] Scheffer RE, Kowatch RA, Carmody T, et al. (2005) Randomized, placebo-controlled trial of mixed amphetamine salts for symptoms of comorbid ADHD in pediatric bipolar disorder after mood stabilization with divalproex sodium. Am J Psychiatry 162: 58–64.

[82] Schwarz C, Volz A, Li C, Leucht S. Valproate for schizophrenia. Cochrane Database Syst Rev 2008; Issue 3: CD004028.

[83] Shaji KS. Clinical Practice Guidelines for Management of Alzheimer's Disease. Indian psychiatric society treatment guidelines 2007.

[84] Shrivastava A, Johnston M, Terpstra K, Stitt L, Shah N. Atypical antipsychotics usage in long-term follow-up of first episode schizophrenia. Indian J Psychiatry 2012;54:248–52.

[85] Smith LA, Cornelius V, Warnock A, Tacchi MJ, Taylor D. Acute bipolar mania: a systematic review and meta-analysis of co-therapy vs. monotherapy. Acta Psychiatr-Scand 2007;115:12-20.

[86] Sommer IE, Begemann MJ, Temmerman A, Leucht S. Pharmacological augmentation strategies for schizophrenia patients with insufficient response to clozapine: a quantitative literature review. Schizophr Bull 2012;38:1003-1011.

[87] Soyka M, Kranzler HR, van den Brink W, Krystal J, Möller HJ, Kasper S. The World Federation of Societies of Biological Psychiatry (WFSBP) guidelines for the biological treatment of substance use and related disorders. Part 2: Opioid dependence. World J Biol Psychiatry. 2011 Apr;12(3):160-87.

[88] Soyka M, Schmidt F, Schmidt P. 2006. Efficacy and safety of outpatient alcohol detoxification with a combination of tiapride/ carbamazepine: Additional evidence. Pharmacopsychiatry 39:3034.

[89] Sung SC, Haley CL, Wisniewski SR, Fava M, Nierenberg AA, Warden D, Morris DW, Kurian BT, Trivedi MH, Rush AJ. The impact of chronic depression on acute and long-term outcomes in a randomized trial comparing selective serotonin reuptake inhibitor monotherapy versus each of 2 different antidepressant medication combinations. J Clin Psychiatry 2012;73(7):967-76.

[90] Suppes T, Vieta E, Liu S, Brecher M, Paulsson B. Maintenance treatment for patients with bipolar I disorder: results from a north american study of quetiapine in combination with lithium or divalproex (trial 127). Am J Psychiatry 2009;166(4):476-88.

[91] Tohen M, Vieta E, Calabrese J, Ketter TA, Sachs G, Bowden C,et al. 2003. Efficacy of olanzapine and olanzapine-fluoxetinecombination in the treatment of bipolar I depression. Arch GenPsychiatry 60:1079–1088.

[92] van der Loos ML, Mulder PG, Hartong EG, Blom MB, VergouwenAC, de Keyzer HJ, et al. 2009. Efficacy and safety of lamotrigineas add-on treatment to lithium in bipolar depression: amulticenter, double-blind, placebo-controlled trial. J Clin Psychiatry70:223–231.

[93] Veehof L, Stewart R, Haaijer-Ruskamp F, Jong BM. The development of polypharmacy. A longitudinal study. Fam Pract. 2000;17(3):261-7.

[94] Vieta E, Suppes T, Eggens I, Persson I, Paulsson B, Brecher M.Efficacy and safety of quetiapine in combination with lithium or divalproex for maintenance of patients with bipolar I disorder (international trial 126).J Affect Disord 2008;109(3):251-63.

[95] Vieta E, T'joen C, McQuade RD, Carson WH Jr, Marcus RN, Sanchez R, Owen R, Nameche L.Efficacy of adjunctive aripiprazole to either valproate or lithium in bipolar mania patients partially nonresponsive to valproate/lithium monotherapy: a placebo-controlled study.Am J Psychiatry 2008;165(10):1316-25.

[96] Werder SF, Preskorn SH: Managing polypharmacy: Walking the fine line between help and harm. Current Psychiatry Online 2003;2(2):published online.

[97] Wilby J, Kainth A, Hawkins N, Epstein D, McIntosh H, McDaid C, Mason A, Golder S, O'Meara S, Sculpher M, Drummond M, Forbes C. Clinical effectiveness, tolerability and cost-effectiveness of newer drugs for epilepsy in adults: a systematic review and economic evaluation. Health Technol Assess 2005;9:1-157.

[98] Yancheva S, Ihl R, Nikolova G, Panayotov C, Schlaefke S, Hoerr R, for the GINDON Study Group. 2009. Ginkgo biloba extract EGb 761 ®, donepezil or both combined in

the treatment of Alzheimer's disease with neuropsychiatric features: A randomised, double-blind, exploratory trial. Aging Ment Health 13:183 – 190.

[99] Yatham LN, Grossman F, Augustyns I, Vieta E, Ravindran A. Mood stabilizers plus risperidone or placebo in the treatment of acute mania. International, double-blind, randomized controlled trial. Br J Psychiatry 2003;182:141–7.

[100] Zeni CP, Tramontina S, Ketzer CR, et al. (2009) Methylphenidate combined with aripiprazole in children and adolescents with bipolar disorder and attention-deficit/hyperactivity disorder: a randomized crossover trial. J Am Acad Child Adolesc Psychiatry 19: 553–561.

[101] Zigman D, Blier P. A framework to avoid irrational polypharmacy in psychiatry. J Psychopharmacol. 2012 Dec;26(12):1507-11.

[102] Zimmerman M, Mattia JI and Posternak MA. Are subjects in pharmacological treatment trials of depression representative of patients in routine clinical practice? Am J Psychiatry 2002;159:469–473.